THE BODY-SIGNAL SECRET

You Know Diets Don't Work. Here's What Does!

By Steven C. Strauss, M.D.,
Founder of the Lighten Up Seminar Program,
and Gail North

Rodale Press, Emmaus, Pennsylvania

Notice

This book is intended as a reference volume only, not as a medical manual or a guide to self-treatment. If you suspect that you have a medical problem, we urge you to seek competent medical help. Keep in mind that nutritional needs vary from person to person, depending on age, sex, health status, and total diet. The information here is intended to help you make informed decisions about your diet, not to substitute for any treatment that may have been prescribed by your doctor.

Copy editor: Lisa D. Andruscavage
Book designer: Stan Green
Cover designer: Jane Knutila

If you have any questions or comments concerning this book, please write:
Rodale Press
Book Reader Service
33 East Minor Street
Emmaus, PA 18098

Library of Congress Cataloging-in-Publication Data

Strauss, Steven C.
    The body-signal secret: you know diets don't work, here's what does! : featuring the six-week body-signal program for permanent weight control/ by Steven C. Strauss & Gail North.
        p.   cm.
    Includes index.
    ISBN 0–87857–931–1 hardcover
    1. Reducing—Psychological aspects. 2. Body image. I. North, Gail, 1939– . II. Title.
RM222.2.S855 1991   90–9096
613.2′5—dc20   CIP

Distributed in the book trade by St. Martin's Press

  4 6 8 10 9 7 5   hardcover

To Phyllis Strauss, whose commitment,
courage, and compassion have had
such enormous impact on so many of us.

S.S.

For Lou.

G.N.

Contents

think, feel, and behave like people who have no problem with food. Conquer your self-sabotage and respond to your Body Signals by using examples of Instinctive Eaters in action.

Acknowledgments

A very deep thanks goes to my wife, Ruth Kadis-Strauss, my best friend and my most constructive critic; to my father, Leon, for his personal and professional love and support; and to my grandmother, Selma Levin, for her endless encouragement—she has always been there to support me and my work with Lighten Up.

Further thanks go to Lisa Serradilla, whose association I will always treasure—so many of us benefited from her commitment and contributions. I'd also like to thank Susan Gredone for supporting the women at Lighten Up and helping them to maintain their successes, and Carolyn Kadis for her work on the original manuscript. A very special debt of gratitude goes to Osvaldo Garcia, Jr., cocreator of the early seminars, who showed me the nature of the problem and encouraged me to do something about it. Thank you, Oz.

We both extend our gratitude to our agent, Faith Hamlin; to our consistently supportive and tenacious editor, Charlie Gerras; and to Bill Gottlieb. We are indebted to Carol, Carolyn, Leah, Sue, Joanne, and Glenda for their generous insights, candor, and valued time. And, of course, to all the women and men of Lighten Up.

Introduction

I believe that if you're a person with a weight problem, you're no different from a person who doesn't have a weight problem.

If you're a woman (or large man) reading this book, that notion must seem absurd to you. You *know* you're fat (no matter what you actually weigh), you *know* you have a weight problem, and you're *convinced* that if you were to relax your vigilance around food and behave like a person with no weight problem, you'd become even fatter. Chances are you're obsessed with weight, and most likely have been on at least 15 unsuccessful diets in your adult life. Right now, you're convinced that the 16th diet will do the trick.

Well, it won't.

But if a diet won't work, what will?

Only one thing: satisfying your body's desires as instinctively as stable-weight people do. It's called Instinctive Eating. An Instinctive Eater eats whatever she wants, as much as she wants, whenever she wants, without ever gaining weight. Why? *Because she responds to her Body Signals!* She learns to recognize these signals—the ones that tell her she's hungry, those that tell her she's satisfied, and the signals that tell her what her body truly wants. It's that simple.

Your body knows exactly what it needs.

To become an Instinctive Eater, *you must behave just as stable-weight people do.* Fortunately, everyone has this innate ability. This is why I'm convinced that people with a weight problem are no different from people with no weight problem. When you learn to behave as stable-weight people do, you resolve your weight problem—not for just a few months, not for just a year, but once and for all!

If you follow the Body-Signal Program, you *must* succeed: It teaches you to return to your natural instincts. And what's the result? You'll begin to behave around food in exactly the same way as those people with no weight problem. You'll develop the same resources and confidence. The behaviors that caused the excess weight to appear will disappear—and, of course, so will the excess weight.

No diets. No deprivation. No self-abuse. No struggle.

Diets are unnatural, abusive, and dangerous. That statement should alarm you. But what's even more alarming is that you probably believe that all of your diets have failed not because diets don't work but because something is wrong with *you!* Here is the proven, documented fact: It's the diets themselves that don't work! Think about it. There's a $32-billion-a-year diet industry out there working to keep you from knowing that diets are useless. But a wealth of documented information on weight control proves it. The most recent scientific proof comes from Thomas Wadden, M.D., at the University of Pennsylvania. As reported on the front page of the *New York Times* (April 1, 1990), Dr. Wadden's five-year study shows that 98 percent of dieters regain all their weight!

Just for a moment, consider your probable experience if this book were "just another diet book." You'd have:

- An excellent chance of losing weight
- A slight chance of losing as much weight as you hoped to lose
- A 98 to 100 percent chance of regaining all the weight you lost
- A 33 to 73 percent chance of winding up *fatter* than you were when you started (as you'll learn, dieting causes physiological and psychological changes that promote weight *gain!*)

Sad, but true. Even sadder, the diet industry continues to thrive by perpetuating egregious myths about attaining thinness and achieving that *one,* culturally prescribed body image. Here are the major myths you've been sold.

- The problem isn't that diets don't work, it's that you failed the diet.
- You would have succeeded and become thin if you had stuck to the diet.
- You overate after the diet because something is wrong with you—not because diets promote overeating.
- You can still solve your weight problem by ingesting low-calorie foods and liquids.
- People with large bodies should respond to food differently than people with small bodies.
- Women stop being attractive when they become larger than a size 6.
- If you are large, you should restrict calories to the point of torture and avoid eating the tempting, delicious foods that others are eating.
- You should weigh yourself frequently, hide food, exercise only to lose weight, avoid stylish clothes, feel ashamed of your naked body, and conceal your needs.

This is the bill of goods you've bought. What has it done for you so far?

The Body-Signal Secret is for the millions of people—80 percent of whom are women—who continue to buy into the notion that happiness lies on the other side of the next diet. The whole misguided concept of dieting continues to keep untold numbers of beautiful, intelligent women secretly feeling powerless and insecure. As long as you believe your body is unacceptable, you'll believe you're handicapped. You'll continue to put critical aspects of your life on hold until you lose weight. And you'll regard yourself as different from women whom you perceive as having no weight problem.

Eight years ago, I founded Lighten Up, a unique program that teaches women to achieve permanent weight control by ending their obsession with weight and rediscovering high self-esteem. Lighten Up is a weekend seminar that has taken thousands of women through a process that graduates refer to as revolutionary—it turns Overeaters who are out of control into Instinctive Eaters who respond to their Body Signals and learn respect for their bodies. The principles of the Body-Signal Program are based on my work as a physician plus extensive research into holistic health, human potential, and neuro-linguistic programming (NLP), a remarkably powerful therapeutic tool. My aim is to recalibrate the perceptual insanity forced on women and large men by the multibillion-dollar-a-year diet industry and help them to reach their optimal weight naturally.

Let me tell you something interesting that happens at the start of a Lighten Up seminar. Right off, each woman quickly checks out every other woman in the room. The heavier women invariably become very resentful when they spot women whom they perceive as *thin* attending the weekend. They view such women as intruders. "How dare these women come into this seminar that's intended for someone like me!" The thinner women have no idea that the others are piqued. Why? They're just as unhappy; they don't like their bodies either.

This odd dynamic is the result of body discrimination and its effects on women of all shapes. Body discrimination has been effective in this country because as women, you believe that if you cannot fit into a size 6, your body is defective.

Crazy? Yes. But what mystifies me is why, with all the women's issues out of the closet, the issue of body image has stayed in! "Body discrimination is like experiencing a chronic backache," one woman told me. "You don't realize you're in pain—you just learn to live with it." She's right. But Lighten Up graduates think differently. They liken their new consciousness to the woman who didn't know that her husband was a drunk for 20 years until he came home sober one night. The phrase, "But I'm too fat!" just isn't real to them anymore.

I believe that the last issue guaranteed to keep you a second-class citizen—the very last—is your relationship to your body. It's the last self-defeating hold that society has on you. Remember that famous "click" of recognition that began to reverberate in women all over the country in the early 1960s? It was a profound instant of enlightenment that stated: "Life has a larger scope than the one defined by your female role." That moment of truth was a springboard into reality. Since then, you've been winning the battle to establish yourselves as equal members in every aspect of our culture. But you have not yet experienced that "click" with regard to the last limitation on you—your body. You're still tyrannized by body image—by weight, size, shape, thighs, stomach, breasts. Real women, beautiful women, powerful women like you are hiding out because you've all been conditioned to believe there's something wrong with *you.*

You must understand that the diet industry doesn't want you to experience that "click" and get out from under that demeaning mentality. Nor does it want you to know how natural and pleasurable permanent weight control can be.

The Body-Signal Program *will* get you out from under and *will* lead you right into that flash of recognition.

It incorporates no torturous taboos. It teaches you how to reach your optimal weight, naturally and pleasurably, and to own it for life!

Here's what you can actually look forward to. You will:

- Eat as much food as your body wants.
- Eat whenever your body wants.
- No longer fear food and overeating.
- Learn to become an Instinctive Eater.
- Never experience diet torture again.
- Begin to handle your stressful emotions without turning to food.
- Shop for the clothes you really want and wear them today.
- Learn to respect your body.
- Drop excess weight naturally, effortlessly, and without deprivation.

I created the Six-Week Body-Signal Program that appears at the end of this book to get you out of your chaotic dieting mess. It's a program that's quickly learned, easily put into practice, and naturally maintained, and it puts you in control of your weight for life!

Who will benefit the most from this program?

1. Those of you who are victims of the diet/binge/diet syndrome. You know you're doing something wrong here but don't know how to get it right—you're out of control and looking for an answer.
2. Those of you who already realize that dieting takes you nowhere—that diets just don't work. You're the people who have given up—the ones who have slowly and painfully become resigned to a false perception of yourselves as being *less* than those around you who have no weight problem. You now continue to overeat as if it were your prescribed fate. You've simply run out of answers.
3. Those of you who don't know the effects of different foods on your bodies. You don't know that some foods may make you fatter, that some foods may produce distressing physical symptoms, and that some foods may boost your energy, while others may drain it.

You're looking for some nutritional answers that will help to stop the eating frenzy.

The Body-Signal Program has demonstrated over and over again that if you teach a person who thinks she has a weight problem to say "Enough!" to the Diet Mentality, that person will become a person without a weight problem and get on with life. (*Note:* For the sake of clarity and brevity, the pronoun "she" is used throughout this book. The principles of the Body-Signal Program, however, apply to men as well as women.)

The thousands of people who have gone through the Lighten Up seminars now unabashedly claim that the program has indeed had a critical impact on their lives—something equivalent to getting married, having a child, or undergoing a spiritual experience. The concepts work. The program works. And we all know it's time.

Chapter 1

The Body-Signal Breakthrough

Overeaters think they must reach their optimal weight for weight to be no problem. They have it backward. Weight must be no problem before you can reach your optimal weight.

In your whole life, have you ever achieved your ideal weight? Try to remember. When you reached that goal, did you believe that your weight problem was solved? If you answered yes, let me query you further. When you weighed yourself, didn't you find the number on the scale still somehow troublesome? Sure you did.

You may have felt a new confidence and plunged into activities you avoided at your heavier weight, but that sense of liberation was fragile and short-lived. Even at your thinnest, you couldn't really keep from worrying that tomorrow the number might move up. To assuage the nagging anxiety, you probably reasoned: I think I'd better cut more calories and lose another 5 pounds—just to give myself a little leeway.

And what about that thrilling morning the number on the scale actually registered *below* your ideal weight? You were exhilarated, but it was shrouded with uneasiness. Surely that number was a signal that you were free to stop the calorie counts and eat out of control again— just for a couple of days!

And, God forbid, when the number on the scale began to move up beyond your ideal weight, you really lost it! Completely unnerved, you plummeted into fear and self-loathing, convinced once again that you were indeed a failure.

As these three scenarios demonstrate, you probably can't remember a time when you've actually enjoyed a complete reprieve from

1

weight worries. Make no mistake—you're not undergoing an Alzheimer's moment. Frankly, you can't recall being free from diet tyranny because even at best, you've never truly experienced more than a rickety peace around this issue. Freighted with misguided information about diets, scales, calories, and control, at some time, long ago, your consciousness got stuck in a no-win weight war. *It's time now to break free and admit that nothing you've done has worked!*

The Body-Signal Secret

This is not a mystery book. You don't have to ferret through a mass of complex material to find where the secret to weight control is buried. It's so simple, it can be taught in less than 7 seconds. I'm going to tell you right up front: *Eat when your body is hungry. Stop when your body is satisfied.*

That's the secret. Yet while millions of people continue to search for the answer, the rest of the world's 4½ billion people effortlessly practice it every day without even knowing it. Even now, having learned the crux of the secret to controlling your weight, you may be intrigued, but you're not satisfied. It's too simple. Basically, you've set your mind to believing that this secret won't help you. In fact, you're probably thinking: "If that's *it,* I've been left out in the cold."

I know that just telling you the secret to weight control isn't enough—it won't instantly warm you to the idea. Although that piece of information is crucial, knowing it simply makes you an overeater who now knows what you're doing wrong but still doesn't know how to do it right. The trick is to become an eater who listens to and respects her own Body Signals. That will take a little longer. You have to learn the how-to of it all.

At the Start:
Shocks to My System

In 1982, I was invited to be a guest at a seminar for women with weight problems. When I walked into the room, I received my first shock. The room was filled with stunning women of many shapes and sizes—from the 95-pound-dancer type to the voluptuous, big, beautiful woman.

As these women began to speak, I received my second shock. They each said the same thing. They all talked about how fat they were—

and how undesirable as a result. Until that moment, I hadn't grasped the extent of this cultural affliction. Here was a problem that no one was doing anything about.

The Lighten Up seminars were founded in response to that evening.

In the beginning, Lighten Up participants eagerly absorbed the new information and quickly began to understand how they were short-changing themselves. But eventually, it became clear that learning to change self-perception was only half the answer. The other half was learning what to do around food and how to control weight. The participants didn't know how to respond to the signals their bodies were sending, telling them when they were hungry, when they were satisfied, and what they really wanted to eat. That's when the Body-Signal Program was completely developed and became an integral part of the Lighten Up seminars.

Figuring that turnabout is fair play, I decided to deliver a few shocks. I knew this program would work for everyone who followed it—without the need for diets, pills, or gimmicks. Many of the older participants had been gaining that steady 2 pounds a year, which meant that in the past 25 years, they each had become 50 pounds heavier. When they put the Body-Signal Program into practice, they found that their weight gain totally stopped! Other participants (of all ages) also found their weight dropping. One woman lost over 70 pounds the first year. People who had struggled with weight all their lives were resolving the problem within weeks—sometimes within days. Their attitudes changed, their behaviors changed, and shortly thereafter, their bodies changed.

Stopping the weight gain or losing at different rates may not seem so shocking until you ask yourself this question: "When was the last time I lost even 1 ounce without being on a diet, being ill, or taking drugs?"

Since that startling evening some eight years ago, thousands of people have gone through the seminars, have learned the Body-Signal Secret, have mastered the how-to of it all, and have ended their war with weight.

The "Numbers" Junkies

The Body-Signal Secret is guaranteed to work for you if you're willing to accept this premise: *Everything you've previously thought about weight control is wrong!*

In my Lighten Up seminars, participants initially respond to this seemingly anarchic information with indignation. "How can you make that arrogant statement? I've been on at least 15 diets and lost over 100 pounds in my life!" someone protests. (Yes, and she gained them back each time, plus some!) Scale and calorie addicts are further dismayed when I guarantee that they'll *never* achieve or maintain their ideal weight if they continue to allow numbers to tyrannize their lives. "I can't live without my scale—that's how I keep tabs on my weight," wails one. "If I don't keep counting calories, I'll balloon up like a blimp!" cries another.

Escaping the Diet Mentality

As an authentic numbers junkie, you, too, are recoiling right now, certain that my statement is espousing heresy. But look closely at your reaction. Your distress demonstrates not only that you're hostage to numbers and their fluctuations, but more important, that you're a captive of the Diet Mentality.

Fat in the Head?

The Diet Mentality is a fixed but false set of beliefs about weight control. Bluntly stated, it says that you're fat in the head! The problem is not your weight—it's your *perception* about your weight.

Skewed perceptions about body size and pounds have literally impaired your ability to make correct decisions about food and weight. It's just not possible to stay thin in the body when you're carrying around a fat mindset. Nonetheless, as a victim of the Diet Mentality, you cling with a fiendish insistence to the notion that the two-step process to weight control goes like this:

Step 1: Starve yourself through clever diets and you'll achieve your ideal weight in the body.

Step 2: When your body is thin, your weight problem will be solved in the head.

You have it completely backward! To control your weight for life, there *is* a two-step process, but it's the reverse:

Step 1: Begin to think like a person who has no weight problem and the weight problem will be solved in your head.

Step 2: When you've solved the weight problem in your head, you'll begin to lose the excess weight without the tortuous struggle.

This is a fact. Lighten Up graduates have proven it over and over again. Once you've fixed the appropriate perceptions in your head, you've taken the first step to guaranteeing that those excess pounds will gradually drop off. It's not a difficult proposition. All that's required to get it is that you reconsider your beliefs and shift your perspective. *When your beliefs and your perspective have been recalibrated, your behavior will change, you'll begin to experience your Body Signals, and your weight will be under control.* You'll feel a sense of mastery over your body, you'll experience a freedom from weight worries, and you'll know it's now within your power to live without a fear of food. I promise you, by correcting the two-step process, a connection will be made that will impact on your life forever.

WHAT THE BODY-SIGNAL PROGRAM PROMISES

When you adopt this program, you will:

- Lose all your excess weight without using "diets," pills, or gimmicks.
- Handle stress without the need to turn to food for comfort.
- Distinguish between physical and emotional hunger.
- Distinguish between hunger and sweet cravings.
- Feel like a beautiful or handsome, thin person before you reach your optimal weight.
- Stay motivated to care for your body.
- Use self-love, self-respect, and a positive body image as your impetus to achieve optimal weight and health.
- Avoid gaining weight after giving up smoking.
- Exercise without *over*exercising.
- Begin to resolve health problems related to overweight (high cholesterol, high blood pressure, diabetes) before you lose an ounce.
- Dismiss nasty comments about your weight and handle well-meaning comments with poise.
- Learn why dieting is a hopeless solution.
- Learn *how* (not *why*) you truly created your own weight problem.
- Learn how to find out what your optimal weight range is, how to get there instinctively, and how to stay there.
- Discover that weight charts are nonsense.
- Find out what foods are really fattening and why. (A hint: It's not simply because of their calorie counts!)
- See why calorie counting is pointless.
- Solve your weight problem once and for all!

There's *No* Reason to Have a "Weight Problem"

In order to develop a weight problem, you've had to go through a host of unnatural manipulations with your perceptions of food and your body. The fact that you've pulled it off at all has overtones of the miraculous! It's taken Promethean energies to put those pounds on your body, because gaining weight is *unnatural*—a negative achievement. What is natural is to respect yourself, to respect your body, and to respond to its needs and desires. When you begin to enjoy a relationship with food in which you respond to the needs of your *body,* I promise that you will always stay at the same weight.

As stated earlier, most of us aren't fat in the body but fat in the mind. The majority of people who perceive themselves as having a weight problem can't make the distinction between what they want and what their bodies want. Understanding and internally absorbing that distinction—not simply on an intellectual level—will pilot you into a totally different consciousness. You'll begin to experience your Body Signals, respond automatically, and begin a new relationship with food.

"Natural" Doesn't Mean "Average"

If you've been thinking that your response to food and weight is average and therefore natural, perhaps this illustration will clear up your confusion. According to some studies, 94 percent of American women dislike their appearance. Because the number is so high, that particular female attitude is considered average. The only advantage to knowing this statistic, however, is that it helps you to rationalize insane thinking—you're able to state: "Well, if that many women dislike their appearance, then it's natural." But that's a misconception. More accurately stated, "Ninety-four percent of American women feel *unnatural* about their appearance."

Alarming but accurate. Now consider these two propositions. Few women in our society *actually* have a weight problem. Yet almost all women *know* they have a weight problem. No, you didn't misread the text. These statements appear to be contradictory, yet both are true. In our rather bizarre culture, the norm is for women to obsess about their bodies. This obsession leads to a distorted relationship with food and forms the basis for the most *unnatural* of pastimes—the reducing diet. That's average!

The Sanity Check

Going on the premise that you function as a basically sane human being in your life, doesn't it strike you as insane that you feel compelled to agonize incessantly over your weight? Think about it. How sane is it to starve yourself into weakness and fatigue? How sane is it to go on a diet when your last 15 diets have failed? How sane is it to stuff food into your body when your body doesn't want it? And how sane is it to hate your body—to look in the mirror and dislike what you see? Isn't it insane to use your weight as the axis on which your experience of worthiness or unworthiness turns?

As amazing as it may be, insane behavior shows up in sane people over and over again. Insane behavior boils down to this description: It's a useful behavior that causes pain and is used in place of a more useful behavior that doesn't cause pain. Bingeing is a good example. Overeaters admit that bingeing may be hurtful, but they insist it is *useful* for many different reasons. They say:

- It relieves pressure and blunts a variety of unpleasant emotions.
- It helps pass the time.
- It's instant gratification.
- It pacifies.
- It rewards.
- It tastes good.
- It's a super narcotic.
- It's celebratory.
- It's fun.

But bingeing also contributes to making you fat, and that's only useful if you need to be fat for a reason.

What would be a more useful behavior that doesn't cause pain? First, it's understanding the difference between what *you* want and what your *body* wants. After that distinction is made, Overeaters are able to suggest more useful behaviors.

- Take an aerobics class.
- Go for a walk.
- Call a close friend.
- Submerge yourself in a terrific book.
- Engage in a hobby.
- Get appropriately angry.
- Take a long, hot bath.
- Make love.
- Go shopping.

Consider this scenario. You're sitting at a desk with a bookshelf behind the chair. Every time you move, you hit your head on the shelf extension. Frustrated and at your wit's end, you finally admit to a friend, "I've had a throbbing headache every day for a year." Your friend quickly assesses the insanity of your behavior and concludes: "Either move the desk forward or change the position of the shelf." "Aha!" you say. "That's the answer!"

As you continue reading, you're going to experience this response again and again. You're going to exclaim, "Aha! I see it now! I've been banging my head against the shelf. There is no need for me to have a weight problem." It will boggle your mind. At last, you're going to understand—"Aha! That's the answer. Now I know what to do!"

And because you're going to be certain that you know what to do, you're going to be equally clear that weight is no longer a problem. You'll know how to control and handle it.

I promise this phenomenon will occur. When useful behaviors that don't cause pain become automatic parts of your everyday life, insane behaviors that hurt lose their power and allure and eventually fade away.

Bingeing isn't *natural*. When you binge, you're engaging in an insane behavior that causes pain, but only because you haven't learned a more useful one that doesn't cause pain.

I can guarantee that when you finally make the connection between what you want and what your body wants, you will experience the "Aha!"—that profound moment of enlightenment. Suddenly it will dawn on you: "What I've been doing to my body isn't natural, and I no longer need to keep doing it. It's the same as hitting my head over and over again on the shelf."

Instinctive Eaters versus Overeaters

The 4½ billion people who understand the Body-Signal Secret and who are expert at the how-to, I call Instinctive Eaters. These are the people who have no weight problems. Their weight doesn't stop them from being fully engaged with their lives, from enjoying good health and a feeling of well-being. They don't worry about calories and scales, food and diets, or use their weight to measure their worthiness.

Instinctive Eaters eat when they're hungry, whenever they're hungry, as many times as they're hungry. Further, they frequently eat more than overweight people do, and sometimes more often. On the other hand, Instinctive Eaters do *not* eat when they are *not* hungry (except on infrequent occasions when they *choose* to eat "recreationally," still in control and enjoying every bite!). But they do *not* keep eating until they're bloated—they know when to stop. There is no mystery here.

They respond to their Body Signals—first, one that tells them: Yes, I'm hungry; and second, one that says: I'm satisfied now. Satisfaction to the Instinctive Eater equals the absence of hunger.

The remaining ½ billion are Overeaters who often aren't sure when they're hungry or when they're satisfied and derive little real gratification from food. As an Overeater, you're aware that you often don't actually know what food tastes like or why you're eating it. What you do know is that you're out of control and don't know how to stop the overeating momentum.

Just like those of Instinctive Eaters, your Body Signals speak to you every day of your life, but either you haven't been paying attention or you haven't cracked the code. They're not complex. In fact, later on in this book, you're going to learn how to hear those signals—loud and clear—and how to decipher their meanings. And the sooner you learn to respond to your Body Signals as an Instinctive Eater, the sooner you'll gain control of your eating momentum and achieve your optimal weight.

Ideal Weight versus Optimal Weight

What's the difference between your ideal weight and your optimal weight? I'd like you to be very clear about the distinctions. They're important. Your *ideal* weight is your fantasy weight. That's the illusory version of yourself in which Tom Selleck look-alikes are knocking at your door and women are staring at you with the purest envy. And why not? You're a perfect size 6!

Your *optimal* weight falls within your perfect genetic/biochemical weight range and provides you with optimal health. At that weight, you're the most comfortable with yourself—and you feel just great! That's the weight that Instinctive Eaters naturally maintain and can call their own for life.

If you are trapped in the Diet Mentality and your ideal weight is out of sync with your optimal weight, the projection is grim. You may continually strive for that unattainable number, but you'll be doomed to a life of obsession, disappointment, and frustration.

Doesn't it make sense to vote for real success? After all, your optimal weight is your genetic/biochemical birthright. The only pounds you need to lose are those in excess of that birthright. Optimal weight is yours for the taking and for the keeping simply by learning to respond to your Body Signals and becoming an Instinctive Eater.

Replacing Your Overeater's Program

To ensure that you know what *instinctive* actually means and how it feels, I'm going to start over from scratch and help you relearn what feels good, right, and authentic to you. At some point in your life, you *instinctively* knew what your body needed and how to satisfy those needs. You had it down, then somehow veered off.

Here's what's going to happen. Since the mind is like a giant computer, you can assume that at some point, someone slipped a floppy disk containing a hurtful Overeater's Program inside your system. You're going to be ejecting that disk and inserting one that's new and different—the Instinctive Eater's Body-Signal Program. The Overeater's Program won't be entirely deleted—remnants will stay in your computer memory. But they won't be easily accessed. As the new program is being "booted up," please remember: You've grown familiar with the old program, therefore, the new one will feel entirely foreign. You may balk and try to dismiss the new menu information, but the truth will be undeniable.

Thinness Is "Everything"

Generally, diet books pander to your insecurities by selling the fantasy of being thin and leading you to believe you're going to achieve your ideal weight. The Diet Mentality insists that you believe that thinness equals an end of conflicts and a beginning of an abstract notion called happiness. But, as Susie Orbach wrote in *Fat Is a Feminist Issue*, "Thinness resolves no conflicts." My experience with Lighten Up participants demonstrates indisputably that underneath the thin fantasy is another fantasy, much more powerful, profound, and specific: Getting what you want from life.

As you continue reading, you're going to stop spinning your weight-problem wheels, move on from that familiar but unproductive going-nowhere thinking, and learn how to actually get what you want. You will discover you can start to make the bottom-line fantasy a reality—immediately—even with the body you're in.

When you're cornered in the Diet Mentality, you like to argue that you can't do anything until you get to that ideal weight. "At my ideal weight, I felt a whole lot better about myself, and until I get back to it, I can't make any moves—I can't have what I really want from my life." Granted, you may have felt "a whole lot better," but the good feeling you like to recall was transitory. As we stated at the beginning of this chapter, if you think again about what it was like for you at that ideal weight, you'll remember that it took more than a thin body for you to continue feeling good.

True, in our society, thinness helps, but not as much as you think. It isn't the inability to achieve your ideal weight that stops you from attracting the men you want to attract, from enjoying the fulfilling sex life you want, from achieving your career dreams, from wearing stunning new clothes, or from experiencing high self-esteem. It's the absence of those satisfactions in your life that keeps you from achieving your optimal weight!

That basic misperception about what a thin body will permit you to do has literally worked against your ability to control your weight.

You're *Not* Different from Thin People!

Given all the schemes for losing weight, there are basically only two theories of weight control. Although the first of these theories is a proven failure, it has been and still is currently in vogue. It states that people with a weight problem are different from those without a weight problem and should behave differently. This theory insidiously implies that people with a weight problem should *not* like their bodies, should restrict calories, should avoid certain foods that other people can eat, should dress conservatively, should make love in the dark, and should exercise only to lose weight.

The second theory is mine. It's actually no longer considered a theory because it's been put to the test and is now a proven success. It states that people with a weight problem need be *no different* from people without a weight problem. The logic works. When you teach a person with a weight problem how to think and behave like a person without a weight problem, *there is no problem:* The excess weight drops off.

Learning to Model Behavior

Through a process called modeling, I promise you're going to learn to think and behave exactly like people at their genetically normal weight. Modeling doesn't mean copying, and it's different from imitation. When you learn to model Instinctive Eaters, you begin to think the same way they think; to believe as they do about their eating, their weight, and their bodies, and to respond emotionally as they do to food. Once you begin to think, believe, and respond emotionally as an Instinctive Eater, it becomes second nature to behave as one. It's a totally natural process that everyone can learn.

I promise you will learn to think and behave exactly like an Instinctive Eater and suffer no problem with your weight.

The Body-Signal Breakthrough

As participants in my Lighten Up seminars begin to build up a consciousness of these weight-control concepts, they suddenly experience a penetrating moment of enlightenment that launches them into becoming Instinctive Eaters. That "click" of recognition doesn't occur because I'm trying to convince them of my logic—it resounds in their own minds only when they get the message, when the ideas all come together.

As with certain peak experiences that change your life forever—getting married, having a child, or for some, having a spiritual rebirth—when you change from an Overeater to an Instinctive Eater who responds to your Body Signals, you will experience what I call the Body-Signal Breakthrough. Not only will you understand what it takes to reach optimal weight, you will also realize what the new thinking means in terms of your entire life. One woman described it perfectly, saying, "It's a wake-up call that comes from within."

It's profound. It's real. And it will alter your life for good.

THE BODY-SIGNAL PROGRAM WILLINGNESS TEST

Consider these questions. If you can answer yes to all of them, you're halfway to achieving your optimal weight for life.
   Are you willing to learn how to:

- Eat when you're hungry and stop when you're satisfied?
- Eat as much food as your *body* wants, whenever your *body* wants it?
- Give up your fear of food and overeating?
- Reach your optimal weight without deprivation or medication?
- Handle your stressful emotions without turning to food?
- Stop using the number on the scale as a measure of your self-esteem?
- Feel the freedom to make love with the lights on?
- Shop for the clothes you really want, and wear them today?
- Master the technique of becoming an in-control Instinctive Eater?
- Finally, and at long last, give your body the respect it deserves?

Chapter 2

How to Prove You're Fat!

If you need to be thin, you're obsessed with nonacceptance.

Allison claims she wakes up many mornings "feeling fat." When asked what that means, she answers: "Large, ugly, bad—as if I'm taking up too much space." Before her feet touch the carpet, she has ticked off the activities to be avoided that day; she can't enjoy herself when she's feeling "too big to be seen." To confirm her suspicions, she instantly begins to amass the proper evidence with which to prove her case. Slouching toward the bathroom, she steps on the scale and flinches (Exhibit A). Not only did she fail to lose those 12 haunting pounds overnight, this morning the scale registers ½ pound higher! The full-length mirror validates the scale's pronouncement (Exhibit B). Disgust snakes through her body. She now *knows* she's fat, and all day long she will be given even more evidence to prove it.

For instance, Exhibit C is hanging in the closet. She can't wear the red suit because red will draw attention to her body, and the black dress is at the cleaners. But if she wears the green skirt with the long full jacket, maybe she'll get away with it, at least for today. While sifting through her "thin" clothes—dresses, skirts, and pants she hasn't worn comfortably for four years—she hears an announcer on television persuading her to use appetite capsules "with 16-hour strength" (Exhibit D). Her belly fills with dread. While applying mascara, she glances up at the set and sees a famous actress finish off a low-cal dinner, whip

13

off a cape revealing a thin, glamorous body, then glowingly exclaim, "*This* is living!" (Exhibit E). Before leaving the house, she grabs her "To Do Today" memo pad and scribbles: "Diet pills—max strength" and "300-cal. entrées."

At the office, Allison calls Dawn to cancel their plans for that night. "I can't go to the party," she says. Dawn sounds miffed; she asks, "Why not?" "I'm feeling *too* fat," Allison exclaims. Her friend's attitude immediately shifts to total understanding (Exhibit F). "In that case, don't worry," Dawn says reassuringly, then adds, "Do I know fat attacks, or what?" They agree to meet the following Tuesday for a film. It's now 9:15 in the morning.

Throughout the day, more evidence to bolster Allison's distress will present itself unbidden. By 9:30, she will have mentioned feeling fat to two colleagues. At 10:00, one will offer her a diuretic (Exhibit G); at 10:45, another will poke her head into Allison's office and suggest a liquid fast (Exhibit H). In the ladies' room at around 11:00, she'll read an article on the skyrocketing trend in body sculpting—flat, flat bellies (Exhibit I), and while turning the pages, note that the ads for lipstick and mousse feature models who not only look like 14-year-olds but look like thin, muscular, 14-year-old boys! (Exhibit J).

To ward off a wave of self-hatred, at 12:30 Allison will take a walk, stop in front of a store window, and check out a promising display of trendy jackets perfect for concealing her fat flaws. Newly buoyed, she'll enter the boutique, but while searching for her size on the rack, a salesperson will inform her that this particular item was only cut through size 9 (Exhibit K).

Although ravenous when she meets two friends for lunch, Allison won't order the chicken salad sandwich she has on her mind. The two women have been discussing calories and will be lunching on diet sodas and salad (Exhibit L). "I'll have the same," she'll announce to the waiter, garnering instant approval from her lunch mates (Exhibit M). She's not ordering what she really wants, but then she can't be seen eating "real food" in front of her friends.

Battling the shame of feeling fat and the duty to "do something about it," she'll decide to make her aerobics class that evening—and hope no one notices her. While changing into workout clothes, she'll listen to the locker-room chatter concerning the merits of tight thighs, taut stomachs, firm arms, and hard buns (Exhibits N through Q). For the next 45 minutes, she'll expiate her sin of fatness by beating her body into submission.

On the way home, she'll stop at the drugstore and the supermarket. The package of time-release, appetite-control capsules will momentarily buoy her spirits, as will the stock of six less-than-300-calorie frozen dinners. (She will not remember when she threw the pint of Häägen-Dazs chocolate chocolate-chip ice cream into the basket.) At the check-out line, she'll glance at the tabloids and read: "Lose 40 Pounds in Three Days!" "Woman Has Jaw Wired for Six Months—Loses 108 Pounds!" "Liposuction Saves Marriage!" (Exhibits R through T).

Waiting for the frozen dinner to cook, she'll flip through the per-sonals of her city magazine and read 22 ads placed by men requesting a "slim, attractive woman—photo a *must*" (Exhibit U).

Between 9:00 and 11:30, while lying in bed in front of the tele-vision, Allison will view at least five commercials for sneakers, breath fresheners, processed foods, cosmetic surgeons, and gyms, each prom-ising a life of fantasy and fun if she becomes thin and rich (Exhibits V through Z). Depressed and demoralized, she'll need "a treat" and re-member the ice cream—"Well, just a few bites won't hurt." She'll bring it back to the bedroom, and without any consciousness of the deed, finish off the carton before the news ends.

Granting Acceptance

What would happen if Allison woke up tomorrow morning, looked at her naked body in the mirror, and said to herself, out loud, "Now that's a damned good body, just as it is! I can be happy in this body. It moves, it breathes, it can take me where I want to go. My God! I love it! I want to care for it, nurture it, encourage it to feel its best. I will never again punish it through deprivation, abuse it through cruel exercise, or allow it to be shamed by anyone else's opinion. *I've had it! Enough is enough!*"

A deviant thought, right? And certainly unacceptable to the prof-iteers of the $32-billion-a-year diet industry who depend on your self-loathing to swell their bank accounts.

If enough of you would say "Enough!" weight-control centers all over the country, which rely on your repeated visits through their re-volving doors, your purchases of their products, and your self-disgust, would lose in excess of $100 million a year!

If enough of you would refuse ever to attend another diet center meeting, drink another liquid food, buy another low-cal dinner, down another appetite-suppressant pill, or feel shamed by your bodies, CEO's across the nation would jump out of windows en masse.

If enough of you stopped despising your bodies and turned your backs on bariatricians ("fat" doctors), acupuncturists, plastic surgeons, spa owners, and legal and illegal drug dealers who count on your self-hate, they'd probably keel over in a dead faint.

And if every woman would just say no to a fashion industry that arbitrarily deems certain body parts to be "in" and others to be "out" (at this writing, breasts are in and buttocks are out), the ministers of style would choke on their spring line.

What would any of *you* lose? If you're firmly entrenched in the Diet Mentality, of course, *you'd lose your right to feel bad about your body.* And if you lose the right to feel bad about your body, what else would you lose?

The $32-billion-a-year diet industry has trained you to believe you'd lose your chance to live happily ever after as only a thin person can. And that would be unbearable! Therefore, you must continually diet your body to "perfection" so you can:

- Stay endlessly motivated to attain a "better" body
- Maintain your future fantasy of thinness (which will bring you a glamorous new career with a skyrocketing income, a great sex life, and high self-esteem)
- Hang on to the idea that if people say you're fat, you're fat
- Go on lying to yourself about your choice in deciding how you feel about your body
- Continue hating your appearance until the current diet (and the next diet) is successfully completed
- Reinforce the notion that you've been right to despise your body all along
- Keep the painful but familiar feeling of hating your flesh and avoid the new and different feelings of being at peace with your appearance

The Skeptic Within

To suggest that you, the reader, wake up tomorrow morning accepting the body you have is not only unacceptable to the diet industry—it's seen as an outrage to anyone who's ever tried to lose weight. When I first explained this concept to Gail, my coauthor, her initial comment reflected the skeptic within every weight-watching woman. She noted suspiciously, "You're trying to make me feel good about *my* body!" As our discussions continued, she raised the objections I run into at every Lighten Up seminar. As she tells it, "Steve's program made perfect sense to my intellect. Nonetheless, as enthusiastic as I may have been about his concepts, they had nothing to do with the private *me*. How could he expect me to accept my body when I knew I needed to lose 15 pounds—by the next morning? Since my early twenties, the subtext of my life had always been losing weight, getting thinner, wearing a smaller size. Like almost every other woman, I was convinced that sacrifice and torture equalled thinness, and thinness would be a springboard to nirvana. Still, his program seemed so eminently sound, I *wanted* my emotions to get involved—I *wanted* to 'get' that impact, to call this piece of wisdom my own.

"The first day at his Lighten Up seminar, I heard my objections echoed back 40-fold. Every participant argued *against* feeling good and *for* holding on to her bad feelings about her body! Although each woman knew she was speaking irrationally, she continued to summon up irrefutable evidence to bolster her case against herself—and the group indignantly supported her.

" 'Why,' I thought, 'are all of us so angry? Why do we continue to lobby for self-hate?' It seemed that as women, somewhere along the line we had acquired a mandate for misery, and we'd be damned if we were going to let anyone mess with it! The notion was unsettling. Why couldn't we see that the bad feelings were *not* a part of us? Yes, my emotions were beginning to get involved, but it was the dynamics that followed that clinched it for me.

"Without any discernible pattern, individual women began to argue *with* each other, and *for* each other—but not for themselves. Barbara told Robin, 'You're smart, you're beautiful, you have a husband who loves you—how can you let other people's opinions about your body interfere with your sex life? If I were you, I'd be wallowing in it!' When Robin returned the compliment, Barbara objected. 'It's different for me, I'm not married,' she said. 'It's very hard to put yourself out there to try to meet men who basically only want sexy stalks!'

"Ellen snapped at Jean, 'You're intelligent, talented, accomplished; you've been hating your job for two years, but won't go on an interview until you're down to a size 10! If I were you and had your talents, I'd be out there tomorrow getting the job I want.' Jean retorted, 'And what about you? You probably could have earned three Ph.D.'s in the time you've spent trashing your body!'

" 'If I were you,' resonated throughout the room until the emphasis veered and landed on the incessantly disapproving culture. From there, prompted by Steve and his coleader, Lisa, the dynamic shifted to taking individual responsibility. The women began to address what they would do *for themselves* if they stopped wrestling with their body shame, and then, *when* they would do it. By the end of the day, too fatigued to fight what had become glaringly obvious, most of us began to respond from our essential selves. 'Okay! I see it!' someone spoke out, and someone else, 'Yes! All right!' The beat had begun. We were now ready. *I've had it! Enough is enough!'* began to reverberate throughout the room.

"Has the voice of my skeptic disappeared? No. To this day, it frequently emerges from within me for a nervous chat, but it now has a worthy adversary to contend with: a new modeling that has irrevocably altered my consciousness."

For Females Only

Years ago, at one of the first Lighten Up seminars, Dana, one of the first graduates, told this anecdote: "Sometime during my childhood," she began, "I decided I was *not* okay and my compulsive eating began. It seemed like something was wrong because I was a girl. It wasn't okay for me to get my clothes dirty, to climb on rooftops, to roll in the grass. It wasn't okay for me to compete, to argue, to be angry, or to be loud. *But,* it was okay to eat. Women are just conditioned in a different way than men," she concluded. "We're a totally different breed."

The "conditioning" Dana refers to is what brings women of all ages to Lighten Up. Their cultural, economic, and political backgrounds cut a wide swath—liberals and conservatives, affluent and poor, homemakers, artists, lawyers, executives, and secretaries. Although the differences are striking, there are three common denominators that bond the group in a tight-knit alliance. Each woman:

1. Operates from the Diet Mentality
2. Arrives with a deeply ingrained Overeater's Program
3. Believes she is *handicapped,* and therefore *unacceptable*

The Woman's Model

I call the last of these common threads the Woman's Model. Obviously, this mode of corrosive thinking and believing has been grafted onto women and passed along by each generation. The fashion industry authenticates it, men validate it, bogus height/weight standards substantiate it. Here are the five stages of the Woman's Model development.

1. You must be born a woman.
2. As a woman, you must obsess over your body.
3. Amass evidence to support your "handicap."
4. Learn to "feel fat."
5. "Do" something about it! Diet!

The Woman's Model isn't difficult to spot—it's exhibited over and over again. Think of the many unquestioned behaviors women have absorbed and reabsorbed over years that produce automatic responses! These behaviors and responses are hard to give up. In fact, until women begin to believe there's another model that makes sense—the Instinctive Eater's Model—women will be reluctant to relinquish what Gail calls that mandate for misery, the Woman's Model.

Here's how the model develops.

Stage 1: You must be born a woman. Much like the succession of royalty, as a member of the female gender, your legacy is guaranteed the moment you're born. Stage 1 is a fait accompli.

Stage 2: As a woman, you must obsess over your body. This stage is launched in childhood. (Nowadays, 4 years old is not too young!) It's only a matter of developmental time before stage 2 gains some momentum and you begin to incorporate your female legacy into everyday life—regardless of your size. Thin or fat, embarrassment, guilt, and "wrongness" nag at you throughout the day. You're embarrassed by your stomach, hips, buttocks, thighs, neck, arms, or ankles. Shame is a constant companion, and the handmaiden of shame is obsession.

Outrageous? Absolutely. Body shame isn't *natural!* Every time you experience it, you must understand that you've bought into the Woman's Model and are perpetuating a baseless tradition. Body shame is a culturally inseminated ploy to keep women of all sizes feeling powerless and one step behind their male counterparts. In her book, *Bodylove,* Rita Freedman, Ph.D., writes, "Our current cultural climate causes a great many women to reject their perfectly normal bodies as abnormally heavy. A body that feels too big casts a shadow over its own image."

The "shadow" is the misperception most women carry with them about their body size. To prove that most women inaccurately perceive their body size, in Lighten Up, we used to ask four volunteers of varying sizes to stand next to each other in front of the room: a heavy woman, usually somewhere over 250 pounds; a medium-size woman, around 170; a smaller woman of 140; and then one of our 100-pound professional dieters.

There were no surprises. They all felt exactly the same about themselves! "I've never liked my body." "I've always felt ashamed." "If I could just lose this stomach." If you search for a corollary between size and intensity of obsession, you won't find one. Each woman *knows* she's fat. How did four women with such diverse shapes become accomplices in nonacceptance? They accepted the legacy of the Woman's Model.

Stage 3: Amass evidence to support your "handicap." Stage 3 of the Woman's Model includes the Zebra Code. It declares: "If everyone around me believes that I'm a zebra, then I must be a zebra." More to the point: "If everyone around me believes that I'm fat, then I must be fat." Over the years, each seminar participant has verbally documented how she has allowed society to encourage her shame, to undermine her ability to live her life *as she desires,* and to insist that she is indeed a "zebra."

The documentation varies, but as Allison showed us at the beginning of this chapter, each woman can haul out on demand Exhibits A to Z to prove the wrongness of her body. Here is a sampling of statements from seminar participants that provide the spine for stage 3.

"The chic little boutiques don't carry my size."

"I won't be photographed next to my sister because she's very skinny—she understands."

"Most of my clothes are too tight. I can't go out until they fit me again."

"Every diet book I've ever read says I'll feel better about myself if I lose weight."

"If I weren't fat, I wouldn't feel so bad every time I read an ad for a new weight-loss technique."

"My doctor told me to lose weight."

"All the height/weight charts say I'm overweight."

"The models in magazines are slender and beautiful."

"From the day we were married, my husband has told me repeatedly, 'Don't get fat.' "

"The elevator man made a 'fat' joke when I got on the other day."

"The construction guys don't whistle anymore."

"I lose authority at work when I'm fat."

"Men who run ads in the Personals want 'slim' women."

"The chairs in the conference room are too small."

"Fat people don't go to the beach."

"The carpet salesman asked me if I was on a diet."

Stage 4: Learn to "feel fat." Feeling fat is now an internalized state of mind, an addition to your other emotional choices. You can feel happy, sad, elated, miserable, ambivalent, at odds with yourself, hopeful, discouraged, or "fat." Like the other emotional states, feeling fat can be either summoned up at will or triggered by outside events. Bear in mind, you don't have to *be* fat to grapple with the feeling. Nonetheless, as Dr. Freedman suggests, "A person who feels fat can have just as many body conflicts as one who actually is fat."

What happens when you feel fat? You begin to behave oddly. You may withdraw, become ill, dress down, avoid dance and exercise classes, make little or no eye contact, blur your image in the mirror/become bonded to the mirror, ignore your talents, apologize too much.

And that's just the beginning; more serious results follow. You may cancel the job interview, postpone the social event, refuse to go to a school reunion, beg off from the dinner date, back off from sex. Summer and premature seasonal changes may also be anticipated with dread: They constitute yet another threat to body invisibility and fling the issue of body shame out of the shadows and into the light. "I won't wear shorts; I need my jackets; I hate hot weather; and I loathe the sun," one Lighten Up participant noted.

Stage 5: "Do" something about it! Diet! An inner environment of self-disgust is now in full bloom, and the feeling is intolerable. "I've got to *do* something!" you bray, signaling the beginning of stage 5. The fix is in. You're out of control! Once you "do something about it," you're on a treadmill for life. You're in the Overeater's Program, and it will be years (if ever) before you can get out.

You go on Scarsdale, then try out Atkins (even though they're basically the same), which leads to diet pills, then a liquid diet, which sends you back to Scarsdale again. You try diuretics, which leads to bulimia (or its trendy offshoot—exercise bulimia), and add laxatives and enemas to your list.

The desperation peaks—you shop for surgeons to suck the fat out and tuck the tummy in. But surgery is a little pricey, so you give hypnosis a whirl, which leads you back to Atkins, then into est, and back again to diet pills. You try the liquid diet "once more," then visit a psychic, and that spurs you to drive to a spa, then join a weight-reduction program, purchase diet books, and rent exercise videos, all of which persuades you to starve yourself into a coma. And, as each something fails, you become more and more of a hermit.

From the Woman's Model to the Instinctive Eater's Model

As you can see, the Woman's Model is up to its ears in unquestioned behaviors and knee-jerk responses. Unfortunately, it will never fade into total obscurity—it will always be a part of your psyche, perhaps, as Gail suggests, showing up as "the skeptic within." Most women have found that it's futile to fight against it. But if you leave it alone and start storing the new Instinctive Eater's Model, gradually you'll begin to alter your beliefs about weight and self-worth. As the Instinctive Eater's Model begins to flow into your consciousness, the old Overeater's Program and the Woman's Model will ebb. The desperation will diminish. At last, you'll have a new, viable program and model you'll never regret having learned. (To be clear, the Overeater's Program doesn't discriminate between men and women, but women experience it as an integral part of their female legacy.)

Fat *Is* a Feminist Issue

According to former editor of *Family Health,* Dalma Heyn, "Our phobia about fat, our revulsion at looking female, our trenchant self-loathing are a scandal. Yet we no longer wish to trace the source of our shame; we are too embarrassed and bored by even a phrase like 'women's issues' to recognize a women's issue when we see one. We prefer instead to battle our own intrinsic femaleness, to beat our bodies into the shape our psyches insist on, till both what we see and who we are don't jibe—just as what society says about the new female equality and how things are don't jibe."

In our society, women hold only 19 percent of the corporate vice presidencies and a mere 4 percent of the Fortune 500 presidencies. For every dollar a man makes, a woman makes 70 cents. No matter what strides women make in business, law, science, or medicine, they remain second-class citizens.

As enraging as these discriminatory injustices may be, they've gradually emerged from society's closet, and some movement is being made to rectify them. But one more bias still hasn't come out of the closet and still hasn't been dealt with: *discrimination against female body size.*

It doesn't take a sociologist to understand that in order for one group to oppress another without physical force, one of those groups must believe it's inferior. That's why it's so critical for women to put an end to body bashing and say, "I've had it! It's over!"

In our culture, the insidiousness of body tyranny shows up when least expected. For example, I'm always stunned when I see display windows on Fifth Avenue that have eliminated the mannequins. The clothes, suspended from holes in the backdrop, dangle from wire hangers and often are pinched in at the middle to portray a 2-inch waist! The message eludes few. "If you're a woman and have any body at all, it's too fat!"

After years of working with Lighten Up, I'm still horrified that women not only buy into this degrading mindset but sell it, promote it, advocate it—and worst of all, live it!

Three Women—Three Mindsets

Leslie related an anecdote that illustrates how body tyranny affects the female psyche.

"I was interviewing for a job to manage a $10-million budget and a staff of 50 people," she said. "The interview was going great until I was asked a standard question: 'What do you see as your weaknesses?'

"I knew what answers they were looking for: 'I've never managed such a large budget before' or 'I'm inexperienced with a staff of that size.' " She stopped here and asked, "Did you ever say something and instantly wish you could reach out and stuff those words back into your mouth? I gave an answer that was completely absurd but painfully honest. I said: 'I could stand to lose 15 pounds.' "

In retrospect, Leslie was appalled, yet she understood why she felt compelled to make that blunder. "We all know that discrimination against fatter people is a reality," she said. She's right, of course. It's been proven that fat people are less likely to be accepted into schools that require face-to-face interviews, they are disadvantaged in job competitions, they are more likely to lose jury trials!

Still, body discrimination exists and continues to persist because women and fat men believe that they are blameworthy, inferior, defective. Leslie believed it—and sabotaged her job opportunity.

Marsha also believed it and allowed others to sabotage her ambitions. "When I graduated from law school and started shopping firms," she began, "I didn't think my weight would be a factor. After all, I don't research briefs with my stomach! But firm after firm rejected me, while students much lower in the class rankings were hired. A few interviewers even admitted to me that my weight was a problem. I finally came to the conclusion that they were right. I was too fat to be a lawyer and couldn't—no, shouldn't!—become one until I lost weight."

That's the rub! Like most women, the authentic piece of Marsha's consciousness knew that her capabilities and her value had nothing to do with her weight. But in the face of adversity, the part that was firmly attached to the Zebra Code caved in. She believed, "If they tell me I'm fat, I must be fat. If they tell me I'm inferior, it must be the truth."

Although Marsha is a heavy woman, Sharon is at least 50 pounds heavier. As you'll see, we need many more Sharons, women who refuse to buy into the Zebra Code, to help change the Woman's Model. Sharon offered the counterpoint to Leslie's and Marsha's stories.

"I was being interviewed for a very important job and knew I was well qualified," she said. "I also knew that my major competitor for the position was a man, and that didn't help. A day after the interview, the interviewer called me at home. 'Hang in there,' he said, 'we're still making our decision.'

"I knew what was going on. 'You know that I'm the best qualified candidate for this job,' I told him, 'but you're hesitant to give it to me because you're concerned about my weight, aren't you?' He was shocked, but he did admit it was true. My voice was even but emphatic. I told him, 'I just want you to know that I will be great in this position—my weight has never stopped me from succeeding at anything! It has never defined me or limited my talents.' The next day he called and offered me the job."

You can't miss the point of her story. Sharon has no interest in proving she's fat. If friends, family, or colleagues tell her they have a problem with her body, she takes notes. She notes that it's *their* problem, not *hers*. Sharon does not subscribe to the Zebra Code. She believes that the only person who gets to vote on her worthiness is herself!

These three separate experiences clearly demonstrate what it takes *to get what you want when you want it!* The choice is simple: You can put your entire life—or even portions of it—on hold until you lose weight. Or, you can start living your life like a person who has no weight problem—and find you have nothing to prove.

Chapter 3

The Damage Done by Diets

*People diet because they're overweight,
but millions of people are overweight
because they diet.*

An invitation to a wedding six weeks away triggered her final diet. Mattie freaked! People she hadn't seen for several years would be attending—people who were sure to think less of her with the 15 additional pounds. "Snap out of it!" she admonished herself. "You know what to do—*stop eating!*"

An expert at losing weight, Mattie remembered that her last diet had proved "successful" only when she reduced her calories to 900 a day. To ensure she would get down to her ideal size 10 by the weekend of the wedding, she got a jump on the hated pounds by launching her diet at 850 calories.

Four pounds came off the first week, and she was (as she knew she would be) in a state of euphoria. The following week she hit the first plateau, gritted her teeth, and cut her intake to 750 calories. The weight loss resumed, and as she had also anticipated, the euphoria vanished: She was tired, strained, functioning poorly at work, fighting for concentration, and dragging herself through the days. "Don't worry about me," she said to her husband when he voiced concern. "Look—I'm losing all this weight!"

When she hit the second plateau, she bravely endured a short series of expected crying jags, and like a sturdy soldier, bounced back into the battle, cutting her calories again—this time to 650.

Three days before the wedding, she woke up in the morning feeling "filleted." But she had lost 14 pounds! To celebrate, after work she went on a shopping spree. That evening, with her husband acting as an audience, she proudly modeled new skinny pants, a leather miniskirt, and a size 10 dress.

A success story? Think again! Eight months later, Mattie had regained all 14 pounds. "I was horrified," she said. "I couldn't believe that all that torture had been for nothing—again!" Then she reasoned, "At least I didn't gain any more weight. Nothing was really wasted through all those efforts except my time." Continuing to rationalize the experience, she concluded, "I basically came out even."

Mattie was wrong. The frustration, dizziness, extreme weakness, crying jags, and overall depression she experienced on that diet (and all her other diets) did *not* leave her where she was before. In fact, within another four months, she had gained an extra 6 pounds.

A year after the wedding weight-loss caper, Mattie showed up at my Lighten Up seminar angry and panicked. "How could this be happening?" she asked. "All my life I've been able to lose weight on demand. But now, if I wanted to lose even 5 pounds I'd have to go on a diet of 500 calories a day! I just can't do it."

You Never Come Out Even

If you're anything like Mattie and believe that you, too, can cavalierly launch on a harsh diet, give it up, gain the weight back, and start again exactly where you began, you must understand that you're tragically trapped in the Diet Mentality. *You never come out even!*

No woman would ever think of putting herself through the nightmare of dieting unless she believed she would actually lose weight. But few people consider the hidden consequence: With each diet you undertake, your metabolism changes (potentially permanently). Those symptoms many dieters experience—weakness, depression, fatigue, loss of concentration, even the "shakes"—aren't for nothing. Diets force your body to undergo changes that distort its chemistry and balance. Even if you're one of those people who never experience those unpleasant symptoms, your body is nonetheless actively changing its chemistry—and it doesn't always cease automatically at the end of the diet! When you chronically diet or fall into the weight-fluctuating yo-yo syndrome, the momentum frequently continues between diets. Anyone who still insists on cutting calories must be forewarned: At the end of a diet, you'll probably come out fatter!

There is absolutely no low-calorie diet that allows permanent weight loss! Only 50 percent of the dieting population keeps the weight off for three years; after seven years, 100 percent have put it all back on.

The Voice of the Dieting Skeptic

Many of you are still not sold on the facts. "So what?" you're asking. "I have an important job interview with some very powerful people in two weeks, and I *have* to lose this belly. I don't care about three years from now (much less seven), I need to look terrific immediately! I've done it before; I can do it again."

It won't work. You may take the weight off in time for the interview, but your body is busily conspiring to keep you at optimal weight. As you'll see below, it's working hard to keep you safe from famine.

"Fine," you say. "Then I'll diet now and then again every three to seven years. I'll just keep taking it off."

Sorry. It still won't work. Each and every diet can perpetuate changes in your body that may ultimately render it fatter.

If you're still not convinced, consider the upshot of this experiment: When British researchers deprived rats of food, they found that the dieting rats became heavier than nondieting rats. Another group of researchers took the experiment one step further and placed a different set of rats on a diet. During the refeeding, these dieting rats gained up to 20 times more weight on the same amount of food as the nondieting control rats. Rodents we're not. Still, like these creatures, while dieting, we also appear to go through metabolic changes that result in gaining more weight on less food.

Some Critical Factors

Ninety-eight to 100 percent of the people who go on diets (or pay organizations to put them on diets) gain the weight back. (That rare 2 percent who manage to maintain the weight loss most likely could have achieved the same results without dieting.)

Of the 98 to 100 percent who gain the weight back, 33 to 73 percent not only gain it back but wind up fatter than when they started.

As these statistics point out, for every 100 people who go on a diet program, 2—at most—will achieve the results they wanted, while as many as 73 will end up fatter.

Genetic Programming Is a Fierce Protector

When you decide to go on a diet, your body and your brain don't realize that you just read this month's *Vogue* or *Esquire* and want to fit into that designer dress or suit. All they know is that they're not getting enough of the calories they want. Your body doesn't catch the drift. It doesn't say, "So you want to lose 10 pounds? Okay. No problem." What it does do is scream out, *"I'm starving!"*

Tens of thousands of years of genetic programming kick into functioning.

- Your body goes through changes.
- Your brain chemistry goes through changes.
- Your emotional responses go through changes.

THE DANGER OF DIETS

Diets can promote a number of medical problems. Among them:

- A form of high blood pressure termed dieter's hypertension
- Congestive heart failure, which can lead to edema of the legs and water in the lungs
- The release of the potent stress hormone noradrenaline
- Diabetes mellitus
- Anxiety and its handmaiden—overeating
- Weight gain in response to depression
- Emotional overeating
- Higher levels of upset and fear
- A higher incidence of family, work, and personal problems
- A greater loss of concentration while performing certain skill tasks
- Shortened life span

In essence, your body shifts into its survival mode (particularly for women, who are the child bearers and have an additional need to be protected from starvation). These changes are all geared to retrieving that lost weight and reestablishing your system to its normal functioning. Your body implores you to eat more than you need, then holds on to as many of the calories you overeat as it can. Should you overshoot your ideal mark, all the better: Now it can provide more efficient protection for the next famine.

What's the result of that diet? You lose touch with your Hunger Signals. What's the result of overeating? You lose touch with your Satisfaction Signals. The net outcome: You lose touch with the most critical factor to weight control—your Body Signals.

Why Diets Make You Fatter

In their book *The Dieter's Dilemma,* Dr. William Bennett and Joel Gurin discuss a very telling research experiment conducted at the University of Pennsylvania. A group of men and women volunteered to subsist entirely on Metrecal, a dietary drink. By pushing a button, the volunteers were able to activate the liquid, which was then pumped through a metal spout into their mouths. None of them knew just how much liquid they were drinking or how many calories it contained. When the volunteers felt satisfied, they would release the button and the flow would stop. Their only cue to eating was hunger; their only cue to stopping was feeling full.

A week after the experiment began, without their knowledge, the caloric concentration in the Metrecal was reduced by half. For two days, the volunteers drank too little, but then they began doubling the amount. Then again, without informing the volunteers, the researcher placed two of the volunteers back at their original full caloric formula. After two days, these volunteers reduced their intake and dropped back to their original rate of consumption.

The lesson in this experiment is crucial to dieters. It clearly demonstrates the body's innate wisdom. When hungry, your body will call for fuel (food) and utilize that food as energy. But when it isn't calling for fuel, and food is eaten, your body becomes perplexed. "What am I supposed to do with this?" it asks. Since it doesn't know where to place the excess, it stores the food as fat.

When you listen to your Body Signals and eat only the amount of food your body is requesting, that food will be used as fuel—you can't gain excess weight! When you ignore your Body Signals—eating when you aren't hungry or eating more than your body wants—your body feels violated and will put on excess weight.

The violation of dieting triggers the violation of overeating.

The wisdom of the body cannot be denied. It has at least eight methods for fighting back against the onslaught of a diet, and rendering you even fatter.

1. Your Metabolic Rate Slows Down

Your metabolic rate refers to the speed at which your body uses energy—for digestion, for physical activity, for replacing and renewing cells, for the smooth functioning of vital organs. When you diet, your metabolic rate is depressed. Every diet you've been on has trained your body to slow itself down a bit more.

The process isn't mysterious. Let's assume that you're accustomed to 2,000 calories a day and suddenly you cut that supply to 1,200. While you're shedding those initial pounds, your body is compensating for the loss of extra fuel by decelerating its metabolic rate. Without even noticing it, you may become less active and spend more time sitting, lying down for a rest, watching television, thinking, and musing about life. Anyone who has been on a cavalcade of diets will recognize those feelings of sluggishness, fatigue, and weakness and will probably remember justifying them as "the price one pays for losing weight."

But even if you aren't aware of these symptoms, internally your metabolic rate is easing down. To hold onto the weight that your body needs, your cellular processes "put on the brakes."

With each pound you lose, the body slows down even further. The more pounds you lose, the slower it functions, until eventually you hit that hated plateau. And with each diet, that plateau is reached more quickly.

Your body isn't as cavalier as your mind. When it isn't getting what it needs to generate the same amount of energy, it busily adapts to the cuts by diminishing the speed of its chemical functioning. With each diet, it becomes harder and harder to shed pounds. Scientific studies have verified that with each subsequent diet, dieters end up losing less.

2. Your Food Metabolism Alters

When you diet, your body doesn't get the message. It doesn't know that you're simply reshaping it through a restriction of food. What it does know is that it's experiencing a serious famine and that it had better start economizing to maintain some supplies for the future. In essence, the body puts itself on a rigorous budget: It squirrels away as much fat as it can and doles it out in energy as sparingly as possible.

To understand how this happens, you might want to use this hypothetical equation. For every 1,000 calories you eat, your body uses and stores 400 calories and burns off 600. But when you launch a diet, your body seeks to hold on to as much energy as possible. At this point, to accommodate itself to the diminished food intake, for every 1,000 calories you ingest, your body will store 500 and burn off 500. After a few more restrictive diets, the equation changes again: Your body will store 600 and burn off 400.

Each subsequent diet teaches your body to become more efficient. It learns to hold on to a greater percentage of what you take in and to burn off less. In essence, by dieting, you train your body to eat less, store more, and wind up fatter.

3. Your Fat Cells Increase

Diets do shrink your fat cells to a certain point—but they do *not* eliminate them. To the contrary, when the diet is terminated and normal eating is resumed, those fat cells not only seek to expand but will also multiply—sometimes even doubling in number. Make no mistake: *These new fat cells are permanent!*

Since the body perceives your diet as a threat, when you go off the diet and overeat, the food puffs up the old fat cells and generates new ones, just in case of another famine. Dieters wind up with more fat cells.

4. Your Body and Brain Perceive Themselves as Starving

It is known that shrinking fat cells trigger a biochemical/hormonal reaction. When existing fat cells are deprived, they release what could be termed chemically based starvation signals that foster an uncontrollable urge to overeat.

A fuel-deprived body can't tell the difference between a diet and starvation. Its natural response is to compel you to overeat. It makes sense that the more time you spend dieting (starving yourself), the more time you'll spend gobbling food up when it's available. And it isn't unreasonable to assume that if you've spent half your adult life dieting, the natural upshot will be that you'll spend the other half overeating.

5. Your Body's Fat Percentage Increases

During the first few days of a new diet regimen, you'll probably experience a rapid weight loss. You may believe you're making extraordinary progress, but don't be deceived. It's not just fat you're losing. Your body is shedding its first available form of energy—water and glycogen. In the ensuing days, the diet will begin to draw from the lean muscle tissue that it needs least. Much of the fat remains.

You might be interested to know that dieting, in fact, is the recipe that cattle raisers use to produce fatty, marbled cuts of prime beef. Like humans, when cattle are starved down, they lose fat *and* protein. What they regain in the refeeding process is mostly fat.

Cumulative dieting provides all the necessary ingredients for an *irreversibly* fatter body, particularly as you get older. Every decade, women convert 3 to 8 percent of their muscle to fat.

Diets change your body composition to a higher percentage of fat.

6. You Become Highly Stressed

You don't need a doctor to tell you how stressful dieting can be. Let's assume you're on a diet and are stricken by another major stress (your child becomes sick, you have a fight with your spouse, you receive a dunning notice for another overdue bill). You're now volleying a double dose of stress—a dose that pushes you over the edge. You need relief—instantly! There's one surefire, quick-and-easy method to relieve at least half that stress and bring it down to an acceptable level—*eating!*

Now let's assume you're on another diet (maybe even a third or a fourth), and this same combination of events replays itself. You'll find yourself behaving without thought. Like Pavlov's dogs, to get some quick relief when those double-dose stress situations occur, you'll unthinkingly stick your head in the refrigerator.

The conditioning is insidious. Eventually, even when the initial stimulus (the diet) is removed, you will have become an expert at automatically piloting yourself to the refrigerator door for instant relief from the stresses of your life.

Although you now understand that dieting triggers overeating, what you need to know is that overeating triggers the release of norepinephrine, a hormone related to adrenaline, the fight-or-flight hormone. Norepinephrine raises your blood pressure and increases your pulse and metabolic rate.

The release of norepinephrine is fine for Instinctive Eaters who occasionally overeat "recreationally." As their metabolic rates are increased, they burn off their extra calories. (Perhaps this will explain just why your genetically normal-weight friends can binge on infrequent occasions and gain not even an ounce.)

It doesn't work that beautifully for chronic dieters. After a few cycles of overeating, the effect of norepinephrine on the metabolic rate "burns out"—it just disappears. But its effect on pulse rate and blood pressure remains constant. That's why continual dieting and overeating keeps you a prisoner of stress.

The biochemical effects of stress on dieters is demonstrated in yet another way. Under stress, people release free fatty acids into their bloodstreams. If you were to take a look at a non-dieter's free fatty acid levels immediately after she has seen a terrifying movie, finished an exercise class, or found out that the boss is on the rampage, you would see high levels of free fatty acids. These levels are the same in Chronic Dieters—at rest! People respond to chronic dieting as though in a constant state of elevated stress.

7. You Lose Control of Your Sweet Cravings

You're not weak-willed when you crave those sweet desserts and treats while you're dieting, and you're not a failure when you finally give in to them and consume huge quantities as if out of control. This is a normal physiological response to the abnormal stress of dieting.

Research has demonstrated that when people are at their optimal weight, the more sweets they eat, the less they want. The medical name for this very normal phenomenon is negative alliesthesia.

But now consider the flip side. Researchers who dieted off 10 percent of their body weight discovered that negative alliesthesia disappeared. After the weight was lost, the researchers resumed eating sweets, but instead of being satisfied with the amount that would have appeased them at their optimal weight, they continued to crave more and more. When they returned to their optimal weight, however, their normal response to sweets returned.

Here's a possible explanation: When you diet, your shrunken fat cells feel like they're starving and want to be filled up again as quickly as possible. To achieve this end, your deprived fat cells move you to eat densely caloric foods—foods rich in sugar and fat, such as ice cream, cakes, pies, and junk food. That's why (as you may have noticed), you've never awakened in the middle of the night craving celery.

8. Your Body Signals Are Distorted

Your Body Signals are the key to the ultimate 7-second secret of weight control: *Eat when you're hungry; stop when you're satisfied.* When you diet, you deny your body's Hunger Signals. When you overeat, you deny your body's Satisfaction Signals. The results can be disastrous and permanent, although reversible through a relearning process (see chapter 9).

A low-calorie diet, by definition, means you must battle against your body's Hunger Signals and continue starving yourself. When the diet triggers you to overeat, the hunger is so fierce, you ignore your body's satiety signals.

Your Hunger Signals and your Satisfaction Signals—use 'em or lose 'em. This means that if you're a Chronic Dieter, you've lost the only tool that absolutely guarantees permanent weight control: You must relearn how to recognize and respond to them.

The Setpoint Theory

There is a wealth of scientific evidence that shows we are each genetically programmed to remain within a certain weight range. This range represents your normal weight—your genetic biochemical heritage. That weight has been termed your setpoint range.

Don't believe the "standards" recorded in height/weight charts—they're totally without scientific validity. *Your setpoint is your authentic optimal weight!* I promise you that when you adopt the Body-Signal Program—when you become an Instinctive Eater—you will lose all of your excess weight. That means that if you are currently above your optimal weight, you will return to your setpoint range.

How Diets Raise Your Setpoint

Diets can have an extremely harmful effect on your setpoint. They can push it permanently higher, and, make you permanently fatter.

Bob, a patient of mine, is a good example of how diets can alter your setpoint. One morning, right after weighing himself, he concluded that the 190 pounds he had been carrying around for several years without fluctuating were just too much. He was heavier than his co-workers, he felt unattractive to women, and he decided it was time to diet down to 175.

He started his diet that day, and after three months of reduced calories had actually lost the weight. Five months later, however, he was tipping the scales at his original 190 again. Much like Mattie, Bob tried to rationalize by telling himself, "nothing lost, nothing gained," but he, too, was wrong. When he regained the 15 pounds, Bob was a *fatter* 190 pounds than he was when he started the diet. He had tampered with his natural setpoint and risked pushing it higher.

The Dieter's First Question

"How do I know what my setpoint is?"

There is only one way to be absolutely certain: become an Instinctive Eater. When you respond to your Body Signals, you will eat just enough food to fuel your body's needs. Eventually, any excess weight will drop off effortlessly. But for now, while your Body Signals are skewed, think back to that time when you fell in love, or started that fantastic new job, or took that dream trip. If you will recall, without paying attention to pounds, didn't the weight just drop off? That was an example of your body moving naturally toward its setpoint.

Another clue to your setpoint range is your current body weight. If you've spent a protracted period of time at this particular weight, then that number may be your setpoint.

The Dieter's Second Question

"If I'm currently above my setpoint, can I diet down to it?"

Only if you want to make it permanently higher. If you want to return to your setpoint and stay there, you must become an Instinctive Eater.

When you diet, your body will respond much like Bob's. The weight will come off, but will eventually return, rendering you a "fatter" person at the same weight. If you repeat this diet/overeat cycle enough times, you'll change your body to a permanently higher setpoint.

The Dieter's Third Question

"Can I lower my setpoint?"

In a sense, people actually have two setpoints: the sedentary setpoint and the regular aerobic exercise setpoint.

Nonexercisers can be reassured about one thing: The lack of exercise will harm only your health—not your weight. However, though there is usually very little difference between the sedentary and exercising setpoints, in very heavy people, it can be as much as 12 pounds.

Most people believe that the more they exercise, the more weight they will lose. This is a myth. Exercise does not reduce weight by burning off calories—it does so by increasing your metabolic rate. But the effect is finite. After a certain amount of exercise, your body will consume more calories and a permanent balance will be struck.

If you're currently exercising to lose weight, that is to say, to maintain your "exercise setpoint," be aware that ½ hour four to seven times a week is sufficient.

The Dieter's Fourth Question

"What if I don't like my setpoint and refuse to accept it?"

If you're a Chronic Dieter and your attitude toward your natural setpoint is intractable, you've doomed yourself to lifelong misery on the yo-yo syndrome. Your diets will move the yo-yo down, but your setpoint will inevitably pull the yo-yo back up. If you refuse to accept that fact of life, you must accept this one: 33 to 73 percent of dieters will wind up fatter than before they started dieting. (For a scientific example of how this works, take a look at "The Diet-Crazed Conscientious Objectors" on page 38.)

Why Diets Are Harmful

Understanding that diets not only don't work but generate fatter bodies is simply the first part of the problem. Diets also cause damage to the body.

Almost everyone believes that high weight is the major health hazard, but there is a lot of evidence to dispute this point. It seems that the real health hazard is twofold: overeating and weight fluctuations.

As I mentioned above, while the diet pushes your weight down and the setpoint pulls your weight back up, you set yourself up for the disastrous health consequences of the yo-yo syndrome.

Consider two women, Kim and Linda, both the same age and both 5 feet 6 inches tall. Kim is what we could call an average American woman. That means, statistically speaking, Kim has spent one-quarter to one-half of her adult life on a diet—an average of 15 major diets. For the last 30 years, Kim's weight has fluctuated back and forth between 120 and 155.

Linda, however, has weighed a steady 195 since age 15 and, therefore, in terms of dieting, is *not* considered an average woman. At her heaviest, Kim is still 40 pounds lighter than Linda, yet scientific evidence indicates that Kim, not Linda, has increased risk for heart disease, high blood pressure, diabetes mellitus, obesity, and premature death.

SOME EVIDENCE ON DIET DAMAGE

- When scientific researchers induced feast/fast cycles in animals, it resulted in a distinct form of high blood pressure called dieter's hypertension.
- In another experiment, swine were put through weight swings and as a result, they developed high blood pressures and heart disease.
- Overeating in humans triggered the release of the fight-or-flight stress hormone, norepinephrine. Chronic elevations of this hormone raise heart rate and blood pressure (which probably accounts in part for dieter's hypertension and its major complication—heart failure).
- After the siege of Leningrad in 1942, when millions of people were forced into severe "dieting," the incidence of high blood pressure quadrupled and was followed by epidemic levels of congestive heart failure.
- Researchers at the Los Angeles Wadsworth Veteran Administration Hospital put obese men on fasting cycles. Eighty percent developed diabetes mellitus. Twenty-five percent of the men died—mostly from heart disease. When that death rate was compared to that of obese nondieters from studies in Norway and Denmark, it was 13 times higher.

How Quick Weight Loss and Fasts Can Harm You

Short-Term Effects	Long-Term Effects
Abdominal pain, anemia, depression and near-psychotic episodes, diarrhea, edema, fainting, gallstones, gout, hair loss, headache, heart arrhythmias, high cholesterol, high uric acid levels, hypotension (drop in blood pressure), malaise, muscle aches	Promotes the yo-yo syndrome, which in turn increases the risk of: diabetes mellitus, heart failure, hypertension, permanent obesity, premature death

THE DIET-CRAZED
CONSCIENTIOUS OBJECTORS

At the University of Minnesota, in November 1944, researcher Ancel Keys, Ph.D., gathered together 36 conscientious objectors, all volunteers for an experiment in semistarvation. The men were all in their midtwenties, of average height and weight, bright, emotionally stable, and anxious to make their patriotic contribution wherever they could.

For the first three months, they were served a normal diet of approximately 3,500 calories a day. Physical activities were required of them, including various maintenance duties in the dorms, plus walking 3 miles a day. Additionally, they formed study groups and attended courses on the problems of starvation. The men were on their honor. Their enthusiasm and idealism about the experiment were so high, restrictions would have been pointless.

After four months, although they still received adequate protein, vitamins, and minerals, their calories were cut in half. Their physical activities continued as usual.

Initially, they were cheerful and sometimes experienced the "high," or euphoria, some people achieve through fasting. But the highs were inevitably followed by depression, leaving them physically uncomfortable and hungry.

Weight loss was quick. After two months, they had lost about half their body fat, but by this time, they had become irritable and argumentative. Tension was so high among them, the group meetings were stopped.

On their own, the men cut back on their energy output. Although they continued the required physical activities, they sidestepped anything extra. They avoided their chores and neglected their appearance. (Many no longer combed their hair or brushed their teeth.)

As May rolled around, they could no longer trust themselves to stick to the diet and had to adopt a buddy system. Cheating was still a rare event, but when it did occur, it was followed by guilty, frenzied confessions. Two of the men suffered nervous breakdowns and left the experiment. Nearing the end of the diet,

(continued)

THE DIET-CRAZED CONSCIENTIOUS OBJECTORS—
Continued

to find some excuse to get out, one man chopped off the tip of his finger.

By the end of the six months, the men had lost interest in just about everything, including visitors and sex. The scores on their intelligence tests remained the same, but they were obsessed with thoughts of food. They began to behave oddly during meals. They played with the food, ate strange combinations, and became very particular about flavor.

At this point, a three-month refeeding began. Their food intake was still restricted, and even though they were eating more calories than they were burning off, they were still miserable.

Toward the end of the third month of refeeding, the men could no longer continue—they were ravenous. In October, the dietary restrictions ended and although they began eating 5,000 calories a day, they still felt starved!

By Thanksgiving, 15 weeks after they had started to regain their weight, they were still obsessed with food and gorging themselves. Their weight and their personalities were on the upswing, but they weren't quite normal. They grew fatter for a while, but when they finally returned to their original weight—to their setpoint—their compulsion to eat began to fade and they began to behave normally.

Interestingly, they did not regain their old muscle mass right away. After returning to their normal weight, it took nine months to regain the lean muscle, demonstrating that setpoint represents the body's need to maintain its fat content, not its muscle mass.

Had the men gone on another diet during this time, as Chronic Dieters often do, it is possible they would have triggered the same responses and continued to get fatter. But since they responded to their Body Signals the way Instinctive Eaters do, at this point, their weight eventually returned to normal.

This experiment demonstrates two essential ideas: (1) How critical maintaining your weight at setpoint is for physical and psychological well-being—even though it may be more weight than you would like; and (2) how diets create the right inner environment for bingeing and becoming "crazy" around food.

Diets on a Day-to-Day Basis

Mattie and Bob are both examples of dieters who learned the hard way that diets can cause irreparable damage. But what would have happened if, as typical dieters, they had continued to seek out the new and ever-available miracle diet?

They could anticipate the following scenario: A best friend who had just lost 75 pounds on the latest round of liquid protein diets would drag them to an introductory meeting to hear more about the ease and simplicity of this new "wonder" program. At the meeting, they would be fed false statistics, such as, "75 percent of the people on this diet kept their weight off a year later." Mattie and Bob would have been awed. No one would explain to them that 10 to 20 percent is a more accurate figure, and that even this figure is deceptive because sometime later, even that 10 to 20 percent are going to gain it all back and probably end up fatter.

Additionally, they would be informed that because they could expect medical supervision—blood tests and cardiograms on a weekly basis, the diet is safe. To top it off, they would be shown a list of short-term side effects and would ultimately decide that risking these effects would be a small price to pay for getting rid of all that weight.

They would *not* be shown the list of long-term side effects. They would *not* be told that this is "just another diet" and that *no diet works!*

It would certainly be understandable if Mattie and Bob were to be seduced into this program. Both would be looking forward to that beginning euphoric high as they watch those first few pounds disappear. But neither will understand that the heightened sense of good feeling isn't occurring because they *feel* good but because they *look* good. Nor will they remember that tyrannizing their bodies into submission results in a shift to irritation, lassitude, and depression.

As Chronic Dieters, they will not only continue to behave differently from Instinctive Eaters, their bodies will respond differently. Unlike nondieters, when Mattie and Bob become anxious, they will overeat. When they become depressed, they will gain an average of 6⅓ pounds—nondieters will lose 5⅓ pounds! They can also expect to overrespond to food stimuli with excess saliva and gastric secretions.

Along with experiencing higher levels of upset and fear, Bob and Mattie can also anticipate a higher incidence of family, work, and personal problems than their nondieting counterparts.

Ultimately, chronic dieting will move Bob and Mattie to incorporate the dreaded enemy of the overweight into their daily lives: emotional eating.

Still, both will believe maintaining the new body they imagine for themselves is possible. You now know that it isn't possible. The evidence proves otherwise. No one can preserve indefinitely a biochemical body that doesn't belong to her! That's why dieters suffer. When you diet below your optimal weight—your setpoint range—your eyes may tell you you've taken the right steps, but your chemistry is much smarter: It knows you're in the wrong body.

HOW DIETS ADD WEIGHT

Your metabolic rate slows down. When you restrict food, your body adjusts to the diminished intake: It uses less energy, which means it burns less fat.

Your food metabolism alters. Your body stores a higher percentage of the food you eat as fat. Ultimately, you gain *more* weight with *less* food.

Your fat cells increase. While dieting will temporarily shrink your present fat cells, eating when the diet ends creates permanent new fat cells.

Your body and brain perceive themselves as starving. When food is available, you feel compelled to eat out of control.

Your body's fat percentage increases. The weight you lose will be mainly comprised of protein and fat. But the weight you regain will be mostly fat.

You become highly stressed. When you deprive yourself of food, you become biochemically stressed and usually feel driven to relieve the stress by eating.

You lose control of your sweet cravings. The loss of body weight enhances your desire for sweets.

Your Body Signals are distorted. Your brain can no longer tell you when to start eating and when to stop. You lose your Body Signals—*the key to weight control.*

Chapter 4

Portrait of an Overeating Dieter

*The more important thinness
is to you, the less likely you are
to achieve it permanently in your life.*

Suppose for a moment that you've suddenly been selected to teach a classroom of Instinctive Eaters how to become Overeating Dieters. (Yes, it's a bizarre idea, but play along for a moment.) Your job is to use your expertise to train this class of people who are genetically weight-stable to emulate your skills. Remember, as a lifelong expert, you're eminently qualified. In fact, as a typical Overeater, you probably know enough about dieting to write your own diet book. (And many dieters have already written them!)

As you prepare your lesson plans, try to focus on the full significance of your preoccupation with weight loss. Think about the topics you might include in your discussions—the dieting, bingeing, worrying, calculating, weighing, measuring, and keeping your life on hold.

Now, how will you begin?

"It's a Way of Life"

You might start off by introducing the three basic premises of the Overeating Dieter: "I want to be thin!" "I'll do *anything* to lose this weight." "Food is my enemy!" Next, you'll want to explain that these ongoing laments are primary, and that only by repeating them over and over again—silently, aloud, to friends, to colleagues, to loved ones, to yourself—will they begin to foster the continuous sense of confusion, dissatisfaction, and desperation generic to the Diet Mentality.

Don't worry about revealing that the morning-to-night experience of every dieter is nothing less than grueling—you'll be on safe ground. But don't forget to explain that without too much awareness, the anguish and anxiety most dieters experience eventually will be factored into their daily mindset as a way of life.

To illustrate just how locked into the reducing experience you and other Overeaters have become, you might say, "Telling a dieter, 'If you feel hungry, eat something,' is like telling a confirmed workaholic, 'Knock it off for the night—get some rest.' They respond similarly. Both will nod their heads, make the appropriate noises, even thank you for your concern, but at 3:00 A.M., you'll still find the workaholic hunched over a tiny beam of light initiating a report on the computer, and you'll still find the dieter randomly starving and weak or bingeing and stuffed."

Let that sink in for a moment. Then succinctly state: "Dieters are as powerfully attached to deprivation as early risers are to morning light or 'fresh-air freaks' to the countryside."

At this point, you may find yourself faced with a group of blank stares. The Instinctive Eaters just won't get it! "Why would you want to deprive yourselves?" one will ask. "Why not just eat when you're hungry and stop when you feel satisfied?" You'll roll your eyes and again do your best to explain: "*Everyone* knows that getting thin is the quintessential goal, the secret to happiness . . . the moment when life begins!" (Expect to be met by an onslaught of disbelief and a lot of chair shuffling.)

Unable to convince these puzzled Instinctive Eaters of the validity of your experience, you may find yourself fumbling for even better explanations, but ultimately, in a fit of hopelessness, you'll excuse the class for the day. *You'll* know your plight is legitimate and honorable, but *they* won't be able to wrap their minds around it. Something's wrong.

Your difficulty won't be hard to target. As a dieter, you can't see the whole picture clearly—only the pieces. Let's face it: If you were able to grasp the magnitude of the dieting distortions, you wouldn't have accepted the job. When dieters do begin to see the entire picture, they inevitably experience that "Aha!" moment of enlightenment we mentioned earlier, and their lives are irrevocably changed.

So let me relieve you of this no-win teaching assignment and get you off the hook. Since Overeating Dieters reveal their secrets to me and to the participants in every one of my Lighten Up seminars, I'll take over from here.

Calorie Smarts

Let's begin the lesson with the plus side for Overeaters and talk about how quick and smart most of you are. Without thinking, most dieters can rattle off the difference in caloric content between a Whopper and a Big Mac, between a chocolate chip cookie and a Vienna Finger. Many can silently size up the ounces in a portion of lasagna, a slice of London broil, or a broiled chicken leg (plus calculate the fat in grams).

Dieters are the only group I can think of who have actually applied themselves to the arithmetic of microwave popcorn. A woman dieter recently explained, "If you buy the plain popcorn, it's only 40 calories per cup. But don't forget, while there are 4 cups to a bag, ½ cup will remain unpopped—so what you end up eating is equal to 140 calories."

Another dieter obsessed with caloric precision enlightened the group on the only "accurate" method for obtaining the exact number of calories in a chicken wing. "Weigh the wing first," she instructed, "then eat it, but save the bones. When you're finished, weigh the bones, then deduct the latter figure from the former and you'll know exactly how many calories you ate. I figure that one chicken wing is about 35 calories." (That same woman is not ashamed to confess that she can calculate the number of calories she ate for breakfast, a midday snack, lunch, and dinner "while conducting a seminar on the theories of modern art.")

To become an ace Overeating Dieter, you'll also be in possession of at least four sources for calculating caloric damage: a calorie guide to brand-name foods, a calorie counter for fresh foods, a calorie compendium to fast-food eating, and an all-in-one manual of calories.

Scale Smarts

Our lesson will continue with an exposé of the dieter's bathroom. I sometimes think that Overeaters don't feel complete without an invisible sign hanging over the bathroom scale that reads: "Make My Day!" Compulsive weighing is indeed the handmaiden of the Diet Mentality. Again, ace dieters may be the only living group who, in the cool light of dawn, can predetermine the psychological temperature of the up-coming day by a number on the scale. Their rituals are important. Most dieters will weigh in only after morning elimination, but some only after showering. Others will hold out until after brushing their teeth. The discerning female dieter always weighs herself *before* applying makeup; the careful male waits until he's shaved. (No one weighs when wet.)

Controlling the scale numbers also takes a high priority. Dieters may complain about problems with muscle tone, but they are extremely adept at easing themselves down from shower rods and door frames onto the scale. They're skittish around uneven tiles and superstitious about sags. However, although it often eludes them, there's usually one magic spot on the bathroom floor that provides the "true" weight story.

It goes without saying that a ½-pound increase can alter the course of an entire day, perhaps forcing a celebratory luncheon to be put on hold, a romantic date to be canceled, a pivotal interview to be post-poned, an entire section of the closet to be avoided.

To dieters, an encounter with an upwardly mobile scale is equiv-alent to a meeting with the Prince of Darkness. They anticipate a day of hellish despair.

Confessions Dieters Are Not Afraid to Make!

While Overeating Dieters can surprise even themselves with their in-ventiveness, they all share a common personal history of frustration, pain, humiliation, misery, and, of course, diets, with every other Over-eating Dieter.

Let me elaborate. When the Lighten Up seminars were initially launched, we used to ask each participant to stand up and recount her weight-struggle story. However, after a few months, it became evident that during this segment of the meeting, the other participants grew restless—even bored. The stories were too similar. We stopped asking for individual histories and instead condensed the two main versions into a simple five-part composite.

The point of these composites is to show that at some time in their lives, most women will perceive themselves as having developed a weight problem. The experience may occur at different stages in their lives, but eventually, it *will* occur.

The Weight Story

Part I: Birth

No Weight Problem

"When my mother gave birth to me, friends and family took one look and said, 'Gosh, this is the cutest, most adorable little baby I've ever seen!' and I was just showered with love."

Weight Problem

"When my mother gave birth to me, she took one look and said, 'My God! I've given birth to a pair of thighs!'"

Part II: Childhood

Still No Weight Problem

"For me, childhood was a time of innocence, joy, and love. When I was in elementary school, I had such fun on the playground with my classmates. I loved my teachers; I loved my studies! My life was perfect—happy and care-free."

Weight Problem

"I learned at a very early age, in elementary school, that when you're chubby, kids don't want to play with you. When they start choosing up sides on the playground, you'd better go some place and hide. If you don't, you'll have to bear the humiliation of being the last one picked and of hearing the others say, 'Do we have to have *her* on our side?'"

Part III: Teenage Years

Still Waiting for a Weight Problem

"Junior high school was thrilling. I really loved being a teenager, experimenting with makeup, discovering boys, going to all those different classes, screaming my head off with my friends at basketball games. It was such a wonderful time!"

Weight Problem

"I loved my life until I became a teenager and entered junior high. I don't remember when it happened, but all of a sudden, these strange protuberances started popping out. My chest and I were a little scared. I thought: 'I'm getting fat! I'm getting grotesque! I'm getting ugly!' So when I was 11 or 12, maybe 13 or 14, I decided I'd better go on my first diet."

Part IV: College
Still Hanging In There

"I got through my adolescence and then college, never worrying about my body or my weight, and then I met this really incredible guy. We dated for a while, then got married, and life was just fantastic."

Weight Problem

"I was very heavy when I was in college and never dated anyone. It just didn't happen for me. My friends would say, 'You don't want to go out with these college guys—they're all a bunch of jerks, anyway!' 'That may be true,' I thought to myself, 'but I'd sure like to find out for myself.' Finally I decided I was going to handle this weight problem.

"I figured I had 15 pounds to lose—I was determined to diet them off. And I did. But gained back 17. The next time I dieted, only 10 came off, but 13 came back on. With the next diet, I was down to 8 off and 12 on. It seemed with each diet I was getting bigger and bigger and more and more desperate, until finally, I became resigned to the fact that maybe I just wouldn't have a man in my life after all.

"At that point, I decided to go for what I thought was my only alternative. If I couldn't have romance and passion in my life, the one word that would come to mind when people thought of me would be *competent*. I would always be extremely good at my job."

Part V: Pregnancy to the Present
What an Oddity!—Still No Weight Problem

"I got pregnant and *gained 35 pounds*. Three months after I delivered my son, I looked in the mirror and saw that all the excess weight had dropped off—without my even having to think about it."

Weight Problem!!

"Shortly after I was married, I got pregnant and gained 70 pounds. But after the baby was born, only 60 came off. That 10 pounds really bothered me. So I went on a diet."

The Diet/Binge Cycle—And Mental Hara-Kiri

And the recitation continues:

"As I said, that 10 pounds really bothered me. But, I thought to myself, 'No problem—I'll just go on a diet and take them off.'

"So I started my diet, lost the 10 pounds, and then declared my diet to be at an end.

"And that's when I decided that my Promethean dieting effort needed to be rewarded by a Herculean binge.

"In the aftermath of that eating orgy, I entered that lofty mental state known only to victims of the Diet Mentality: Mental Hara-Kiri."

So far, our composite Overeater's story is simple enough for anyone to follow. But only fellow dieters will immediately recognize that altered state of consciousness—Mental Hara-Kiri—and its self-berating litany: "How could I have eaten that?" "I hate myself; I hate my body; I hate this flesh." "I'm out of control!" "I'm weak-willed!" "My God, I'm so stupid, so ugly!" "I think I'm going crazy!" "I can't wear these pants; I can't wear that dress; I can't wear red; I can't wear white; I can't cut my hair; I can't tuck this shirt in; I can't be seen . . . Oh, God!" The chant is repeated again and again until the dieter morally, spiritually, and emotionally kills herself off. At that point, she knows what she must do—return to the diet.

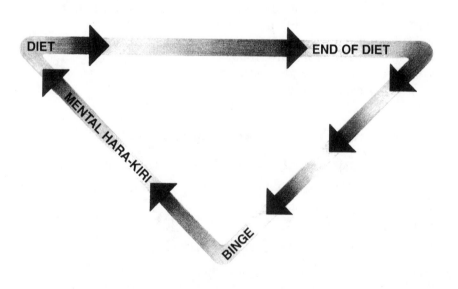

But this time, our composite dieter experiences a hitch in the pattern. She doesn't quite arrive at the end of the diet before she finds herself interrupting its tortuous momentum with, yes—the binge.

Now at binge, she moves directly to Mental Hara-Kiri. And from Mental Hara-Kiri back to diet. And from diet back to binge. And from binge back to Mental Hara-Kiri, at which point she says, "This is too tedious—let's streamline it."

This time, she bypasses diet altogether and heads directly for binge—and back to Mental Hara-Kiri—and back to binge—and back to Mental Hara-Kiri, yo-yoing ad nauseam.

Again, she grows tired of this repetitious game and now decides to add some creative flourishes. In time, a portrait develops that winds up looking something like this:

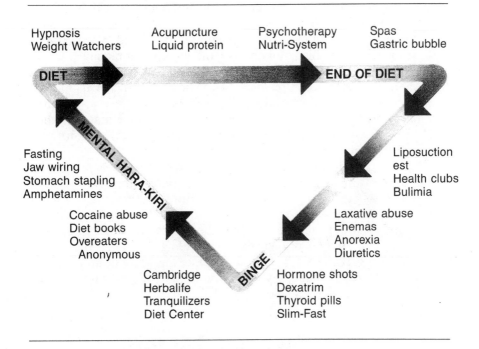

She entitles this portrait of her dieting life "The Mess."

Eccentricities, Quirks, and Hunger

At this point in our lesson, the classroom of Instinctive Eaters will have their collective jaws dropping in shock and disbelief. Not so for any

Overeating Dieters who might be listening in. Their response would be, "Doesn't sound strange to me!"

Overeating Dieters already know that their fellow victims of the Diet Mentality engage in these practices. What they don't know, however (because they never wanted to admit it—even to each other), is that much of what they consider their "secret, quirky behavior," is also commonly practiced by every other dieter.

Overeaters frequently feel that the ways in which they privately behave around food touches on the deviant. Sadly, it's safe to say that all Overeaters feel shame over their weight, and many feel shame over their hunger. It's as if hunger equals badness. And when Overeaters observe their own quirky behaviors around food, their shame is compounded. They're certain that because they engage in what they think are deviant food acts, something must be wrong with them. They fear that they must have some type of psychological defect, weakness of will, or serious character flaw.

Unfortunately, they never were shown the World War II starvation studies and the bizarre behavior the conscientious objectors exhibited who participated in that experiment (see "The Diet-Crazed Conscientious Objectors" on page 38). They never learned that unconventional behavior around food is a physiological response to hunger and deprivation. They were never told that those who ignore their Body Signals and diet, and who drop their weight below setpoint, will exhibit the same quirky behaviors.

To get past the shame, in Lighten Up seminars, I ask the participants to 'fess up. Overeaters would never confess these practices to civilians (their term for the genetically thin), but they know they're safe in this setting. When they hear that their overeating brothers and sisters are also living out their secrets, the shame evaporates. Laughter takes over. As a matter of fact, they often congratulate each other on their creativity. Some even begin to feel like members of an exclusive club—a club that includes several million fellow dieters and excludes 4½ billion Instinctive Eaters.

Confessions Dieters Were Afraid to Make

To complete your lesson, members in good standing with the Overeater's Club have agreed to share some of their rites and rituals.

Unfinished Business: The Leftovers

"I had second thoughts about that pepperoni pizza I threw in the garbage, so I went back after it!"

"My family thinks I'm wonderful because I always jump up and take their plates into the kitchen to clean them off. They still don't know the leftover chicken and potatoes go into my mouth."

"I can't bring myself to throw good food into the garbage. I figure it's better to throw it into the garbage can between my lips!"

"When I clear my guests' plates—I *clear* my guests' plates!"

The Main Artery: Grocery Stores

"If I buy a week's groceries, I don't have to put them away. The entire supply is gone within an hour of my arriving home."

"I plan my shopping around the grocery store's food demonstrations—you know, where they give away free samples of candies or cookies or cheese or crackers or lunch meat or . . . ."

"It's common for me to throw potato chips, cherry Danish, Oreos, chocolate kisses—a lot of good stuff—into my shopping cart and, as I'm being checked out, comment on the number of guests who are coming for three days."

"If I get hungry while I'm shopping, I'll grab some refrigerated cookie dough and eat it raw while I'm walking through the aisles."

"I've left my house in a bona fide hurricane to stock up on banana cake and rocky road ice cream."

Other People's Homes, Other People's Food

"When I'm at a friend's house, I'll go through her refrigerator and swipe food."

"I've made it a point to visit particular friends because I knew their refrigerators and cupboards were stocked with candy bars, ice cream, chopped liver, pita bread, nacho chips—all the terrific food I can't have around me!"

"I've taken food gifts (that I love) to friends so I could have an excuse to eat some."

Takeout and Delivery

"I've bought four Big Macs, four large fries, three milk shakes, and a regular coffee from McDonald's and pretended it was for a group."

"I've called for an extra-large meatball pizza to be delivered. When the buzzer rang, I've turned on the shower, then opened the door and yelled to the bathroom, 'Hurry up, Joe! The pizza's here!' "

Eating Out

"I've gone to three lunches and two dinners in one day."

"I've ordered a salad—or something I really didn't want, so the other people wouldn't know I loved food—then went home and ate the refrigerator."

"I've brought home a doggie bag and, as soon as the door closed, ate the entire contents plus a Kraft macaroni and cheese dinner that was in the cupboard."

"I've eaten dinner before going out to dinner on a date so I wouldn't appear too hungry."

"If you really want to get my goat, go to dinner with me, order the same meal, and get the larger portion!"

Home Lies

"I've finished off three-quarters of a large pork roast, then told my husband it had gone bad and I had to throw it out."

"To make sure of getting enough to eat, I've given my husband smaller portions than myself."

"I've eaten chocolate chocolate chip ice cream from the top of the carton, then smoothed it out to make it look untouched."

"I've eaten chocolate chunk ice cream from the bottom of the carton so it wouldn't be noticed."

"I've eaten a whole carton of chocolate ripple ice cream, then raced out to the supermarket to replace it."

"I've hidden M&M's, Hershey bars, and candy kisses under the bed, in the washing machine, in shoe boxes—then forgotten where I put them."

"I've said I was going to church, then snuck off to eat."

"I thought I was really low when I framed my children, but I found a way to sink even lower: I framed my pet! Get what I mean?!"

Food Obsessions

"If I am what I eat, I must be a meatball hero!"

"I can't get into bed at night without bringing food in with me."

"I watch the clock for my next snack."

"I think so much about food that when I actually get around it, I'm ashamed. Everyone must know! It's like I'm a dirty old man!"

"I worry that my child will get too fat."

"You! I worry that my child will *catch* my fat!"

"I keep all my clothes from my thinner days in front of the closet to remind me of where I should be and to keep me humble lest I forget!"

"I worry that my husband will get thin and leave me."

"I worry that my wife will get thin and leave me."

"I worry that if I lose this weight, my husband will leave me—or I'll leave him."

"I worry that if I lose this weight, I'll leave my wife."

The Nightmare of Overeaters

Now you understand why you cannot teach an Instinctive Eater to become an Overeating Dieter. The training would be more grueling than the Marines' boot camp.

To become an Overeating Dieter, you must be adept at the fine art of starving, stuffing, and suffering. Being a pro means you also feel deprived when you're not dieting and that the obsessions of the Diet Mentality will continue indefinitely throughout your life.

Huge portions of your life will be spent thinking about food. Even when you are not thinking about it, you will be thinking about it! Perhaps at work, while preparing an exciting ad campaign, you will be thinking about lunch. Possibly while making love, you will be thinking about what to snack on when you're finished. While shopping for clothes, you may be thinking about the foods you won't eat. While walking, sitting, playing chess, or hailing a cab, you could be worrying about the effects of the food you just ate, what you will order when you do eat, or how to avoid the food that might become available to eat. Your consciousness can be so completely preoccupied with food that paradoxically, when you do put a forkful into your mouth, you won't even be aware enough of the delicious taste, the smell, and the texture to enjoy the experience.

Intermittently, you'll lash out and ravish the freezer. In the aftermath, you'll feel defeated, worthless, disgusting, vile. Often you'll feel crazed, as if stuck in a nightmare that has no end.

With no exit at hand, you'll finally blurt out: "How do I get out of this mess?"

I'm about to hand you the key.

Chapter 5

The Secrets of Instinctive Eaters

Doing the things that make life great gives you the emotional tools to become an Instinctive Eater.

You now know that you're caught in the diet cycle nightmare, but how are you going to get out of this mess? By learning the secrets of Instinctive Eaters—the thinking, behavior, and beliefs of those 4½ billion people who respond to their Body Signals and effortlessly maintain a stable weight.

As these secrets are revealed, you're going to be coached in the how-to of handling common stressful situations that frequently stump beginning Instinctive Eaters. Through a series of "Miniscripts to Change Your Life," you'll be an eyewitness to the responses of an Instinctive Eater versus a Chronic Dieter in action, and literally see how differently each thinks, feels, and behaves. By the end of this chapter, you'll be ready to begin modeling Instinctive-Eater behavior, confident that you're in control of your body and your weight.

Instinctive Eaters and Overeaters: The Critical Difference

Let me begin with an important definition: Instinctive Eaters are people who love themselves. Out of loving themselves, they love their bodies;

out of loving their bodies, they eat when they're hungry and stop when they're satisfied. (It's that simple!)

There is one critical difference that separates what people who instinctively maintain a stable weight *do* and what Overeaters *do*.

Again—people who instinctively maintain a stable weight almost always eat when their bodies are hungry and stop when they're satisfied—that's it!

Overeaters, on the other hand, act out three variations on this theme.

1. They eat when their bodies are not hungry.
2. They do not eat when their bodies are hungry (*i.e.,* they diet).
3. They eat when their bodies are hungry and then continue eating beyond satisfaction.

That's all you really need to know to become an Instinctive Eater. But simply knowing what separates you from them isn't enough.

It's also worth noting that many body types can't handle sugar, white flour, alcohol, and junk food without gaining weight. To become an Instinctive Eater, you also have to learn to *control*—not necessarily eliminate—your intake of these items. (You'll read about this in chapter 11.)

Instinctive Thinking

At the beginning of each of my seminars, the critical difference between Instinctive Eaters and Overeaters is thoroughly explained, followed by a clear and succinct announcement: "In order to control your weight permanently, all you have to *do* is eat when your body is hungry, stop when it's satisfied, and control your intake of processed foods."

The secret is out. Still, no one in the group actually feels that her weight problem has been solved. It's too early. Toward the end of the seminar, however, when that announcement is repeated, the group sense has completely changed to one of satisfaction. At this point, everyone feels certain that they will, in fact, do what they need to do to control their weight permanently.

Why does it take so long (in my seminars, two days of intensive work) to absorb the basic secret of Instinctive Eaters? Doing what it takes to change from an Overeater to an Instinctive Eater requires a change in *thinking*. Before you can *act* as an instinctively stable-weight person, you have to learn to *think* like one. *Before you can solve the weight problem in your body, you must solve the weight problem in your mind.* Again, you can't achieve normal weight in your body if you're still fat in your head!

Seminar participants learn to respond instinctively to their Body Signals by first absorbing the secrets of instinctive *thinking.* The process begins by making two radical changes in attitude. I call these changes the principles of No Voting and It's My Choice. Let me explain.

The Secret of "No Voting"

There will always be people in your life who will insist that you look and behave according to their tastes. These people have the ability to tyrannize Chronic Dieters, to make them feel even worse about themselves. Victims of the Diet Mentality are extremely susceptible to the judgments of others—it goes with the territory. They're more dependent on others for making decisions and forming opinions than nondieters are. For instance, a compliment or a criticism will inevitably sway a dieter's self-appraisal. Rather than rely on their own internal resources, Chronic Dieters become subject to the whims of their environment. In a nutshell, they feel their own judgments are shaky. As a result, they relinquish their power and allow others to vote on their appearance and behavior.

For Chronic Dieters, adopting the principle of No Voting is essential. Scientific studies have demonstrated that the loss of judgment in one area inevitably spins out and affects other areas of your life—areas not necessarily related to food and weight. As a Chronic Dieter, you now know that you've lost touch with your Hunger/Satisfaction Body Signals. But you may not know that your ability to judge when and how to eat has also been lost in the diet/binge scuffle—and eating when you're hungry is critical to controlling weight. *It's virtually impossible to learn to respond to your Body Signals when your actions are determined by external influences!* If you continue to be seduced by opinions, ideas, and time schedules of others, you'll continue to allow them to vote on who you are.

For Instinctive Eaters, on the other hand, No Voting is second nature. They allow other people to have their preferences, but they simply would never allow anyone—lovers, friends, or strangers—to impose those preferences on their lives. Instinctive Eaters know how to discourage all attempts by others to vote on their appearance or their behaviors.

Miniscripts to Change Your Life

To give you an even clearer picture of how differently Instinctive Eaters and Overeaters respond, try to imagine a set of twins—we'll call them Nancy and Carol. This unlikely pair leads identical lives, their only difference being one of attitude. Nancy is a Chronic Dieter firmly ensnared in the Diet Mentality who continues to respond to other people's preferences. Her sister, Carol, is much luckier. She has just graduated from my seminar and has become an Instinctive Eater who responds to her Body Signals.

In each of the following scenes, the two women are confronted with stressful voting situations. In the "Reaction," you'll see the way each responds and you'll get a better idea of how No Voting works.

Scene I

Handling Insensitive Comments

Dressed up for an evening out, Nancy and Carol are standing with their dates inside a charming little restaurant, waiting for the maître d' to seat them. The men turn to the twins and remark, "You look great tonight!" Nancy and Carol smile appreciatively, but one of the men adds, "You know, I recently read an article on fitness that said there's no such thing as spot reducing. Too bad. If you could just lose that extra fat on your thighs, you would be perfect."

Reaction

Nancy *Chronic Dieter*	Carol *Instinctive Eater*
She does her best to control the expression on her face, which is now betraying a quick transformation from buoyancy to deflation. Just a minute ago, she was feeling extremely attractive; now she feels much like a sack of potatoes. "Yes," she murmurs, "my thighs *do* ruin my body." Despite the fact that she is hungry, Nancy orders a simple salad, hoping to convey the message, "See, I am really not a 'piggy' person."	She looks him in the eye and, like a teacher explaining a concept to a slow student, says, "This is a *perfect* body. As a matter of fact, I'll bet this is *the* most perfect body you've ever been out with! Now, can we just get that table over there and enjoy our dinner?" Carol orders anything on the menu that appeals to her that night.

Nancy is always defensive about her figure. She even overlooks the bad manners that led her escort to make such a rude remark because she feels sure he's right! Carol, on the other hand, knows a nasty crack when she hears one, and she doesn't let it go by without setting the record straight. She is in charge of judging her thighs.

Scene II

Handling Rude People

This time, the twins are dressed in running shorts, jogging in place on a street corner while waiting for a traffic light to change. A sleazy guy now approaches them, points to their backsides, and sneers, "Is that all yours?"

Reaction

Nancy	Carol
Chronic Dieter	*Instinctive Eater*

Humiliated, Nancy runs a full block to remove herself from the terrible scene, then slouches toward home. "I must be an idiot to let myself be seen in public in these shorts with *this* bottom! This is the last time I'll let myself be insulted on the street. How depressing! I need a good binge, and tomorrow, I'm starting a strict diet!"

"That's incredible," Carol thinks. "This guy has such a sewer for a mind—is that all he can think of to say to me? Oh, well, I can't concern myself with every social idiot I encounter." She continues her run and quickly puts the incident out of her mind.

As you can see, Carol, our representative Instinctive Eater, brooks no interference with her sense of self. She will not allow anyone but herself to vote on her appearance or to influence what she knows is right for her body.

The Secret of "It's My Choice"

The second radical change that victims of the Diet Mentality must undergo to become Instinctive Eaters is to chuck the belief that fate controls their lives. Chronic Dieters don't believe that they have the power to choose or that they've actively chosen to feel and to be the way they are. "I just *feel* the way I feel" and "I just *am* the way I am" are two commonly repeated statements. The idea of free will may have merit to Chronic Dieters in the abstract, but when it comes to the personal—how they view themselves—it's usually discredited. The most intelligent dieters have trouble understanding that upon waking, they set up their day by making one (or all) of the following statements to themselves.

"Today I choose to have low self-esteem."
"Today I choose to dislike some of my body parts."
"Today I choose to believe that people who make negative comments about my weight are right."
"Today I choose to find my body repulsive."
"Today I choose to be obsessed with thinness."
"Today I choose to feel bad about who I am and how I look."
"Today I choose to eat out of control."
"Today I choose not to be an exerciser."

It's not easy for Chronic Dieters to admit that these responses are actively chosen and that there *is* another way to think and feel. They believe these responses are natural and therefore carved in granite. Their arguments for the right to feel bad are fiercely justified, as in this typical statement:

It's unfortunate, but it just so happens that given my weight and other faults, I am a person with naturally low self-esteem. It comes from my *objectively* ugly body that *unquestionably* should be thinner with fewer fat-and-ugly bulges, which are so *deservedly* an object of criticism and disgust by others and for which any sane, reasonable person would, of course, feel bad.

Instinctive Eaters think this is crazy! They just don't get it. They would never choose such a skewed perspective on their bodies or choose to beat themselves up with self-abusive language or choose to expect criticism and rejection as a way of life. They choose to feel good about themselves, to celebrate new opportunities, to volley sticky situations with humor—and then to forget them. Here's how these choices are scripted.

Scene III

The Beach Party

Pam, a colleague from the office, phones Nancy and Carol to invite them to her beach club for a party to which the entire staff has been invited.

Reaction

Nancy	Carol
Chronic Dieter	*Instinctive Eater*
She replies, "Pam, you must be joking! I work with those people. I'd be humiliated! Do you think I'd have the bad taste to show my fat in a bathing suit? I'd lose their complete respect! Invite me next year, after I've lost 20 pounds."	She replies, "What fun—what a great idea! I can't wait! What time? And how do I get there?"

Scene IV

Handling "Supposed" Comparisons

In this scene, Nancy and Carol are standing on the street talking to their boyfriends when a tall, slender blond walks past. The men ogle her, then remark, "Now that's one sexy woman!"

Reaction

Nancy	Carol
Chronic Dieter	*Instinctive Eater*
As she eyes the blonde, she immediately feels inadequate, envious, and diminished. She begins to withdraw.	Laughing, she coquettishly whispers, "And here's another very sexy woman—*right?!*"

As you can see, Nancy believes she has no choice in how she will finesse this predicament and resorts to old knee-jerk responses. Conversely, Carol automatically defines her own reality, choosing to get the good out of each situation.

The Secret of Thinking You're Fine the Way You Are

If you are an Overeating Dieter, like Nancy, you probably see yourself often as flawed and unworthy. You do not believe that you have any control over that vision—it is simply just the way you feel. The notion that you have a choice may never have occurred to you.

Ultimately, we all choose how we see ourselves. We're the ones who define, then interpret, our own reality. Our thoughts, beliefs, and feelings are self-selected! To a victim of the Diet Mentality, it feels "natural" to choose suffering, to choose isolation, to choose to heckle and torture herself with irrational messages of self-disgust.

Now think of it this way: Isn't it basically a self-indulgent task to needlessly produce feelings of anxiety and worthlessness in yourself? It's exceedingly easy to manufacture and legitimize put-downs and castigations and then to pass them off as "natural."

New Instinctive Eaters have learned that wallowing in familiar self-inflicted pain is an irresponsible response to life. They're aware that remaining tethered to a negative self-image means they have abdicated responsibility for their own choices—for their own well-being.

Up to this point, it's been rather easy for you to give up by giving in to self-defeating choices. Your reason for refusing to choose to think you're fine the way you are has an ironic twist. To you, the lie feels like the truth and the truth feels like a lie.

Let me be more specific.

The lie—you are fat, unattractive, and unworthy—feels right.

The truth—you are beautiful and important without having to change—feels wrong.

But now, as you tuck more secrets of Instinctive Eaters under your belt, you're going to get rid of that twist. You're going to begin to deprogram yourself by dumping the old propaganda. You're going to begin to see the truth of your reality and make some new, life-enhancing choices. Think about it. What if you really *choose* to live as if you believe the truth? It will change your life.

At first, the new perspective will take a little practice. Fake it, if you must, but stay with it—and stay conscious! Try to catch the lies you tell yourself as they're happening. Before long, you'll notice that your thinking has actually changed, that your new view of yourself—internal and external—has become real, even routine. Take a moment and study the following scene.

Scene V

The Health Club

The twins have just entered their new health club. Both are feeling somewhat exuberant at the idea of plunging into some serious exercise and getting into better shape. At that moment, they notice two full-size, backlit photographs of Cher and Raquel.

Reaction

| **Nancy** | **Carol** |
| *Chronic Dieter* | *Instinctive Eater* |

Nancy (*Chronic Dieter*)

She chooses to see them as "better" than herself and gets that sinking feeling in the pit of her stomach. "Wow! They're so thin and gorgeous," she thinks. "What's the point of trying? I'll never look like that." Depressed and deflated, she loses her enthusiasm and does a only fraction of the exercise she had intended to do. Worse, she gets no sense of satisfaction from the workout.

Carol (*Instinctive Eater*)

She laughs aloud, then says to herself, "Are they kidding? They can't seriously expect me to look like that! Skinny and firm is beautiful for some, but so is *round and firm*. And that's why I'm here!" After a moment, her mood changes to indignation as she thinks, "What are we women doing to ourselves? Why do we all believe we should look like these skinny actresses? Boy! Have we been brainwashed! Our role models are one woman who's had multiple plastic surgeries and another who's had her 12th ribs surgically removed to give her a smaller waist!"

Notice how Nancy continues to buy into the propaganda of the Diet Mentality, while Carol stands firm on her own perceptions. Like the truth-seeker in *The Emperor's New Clothes*, Carol will not allow group choices to distort her perceptions.

The Secret of Saying No and Yes at Mealtime

No Voting and It's My Choice play important roles in the fiascoes Chronic Dieters have made of mealtimes. There are myriad excuses you manufacture to eat when you're not hungry and to not eat when you are. Instinctive Eaters never allow others to vote on their timetables or to choose what they will eat. They have one and only one measure for saying no or yes to food—their Body Signals.

Scene VI

Dinner at Grandma's House

Pushing back from the dinner table, Nancy and Carol both soothe their obviously full stomachs with their hands. Grandma beams as she hears them remark, "What a great dinner! I haven't been this stuffed in a long time."

Glowing with pleasure, their grandmother smiles. "Now comes the best part," she says as she walks back into the kitchen, then emerges with a plate holding a double-fudge chocolate cake. "This was always your favorite," she remarks. "I spent hours baking this treat just for you."

"Oh, Grandma, I'm too stuffed!" the twins both reply.

"Nonsense," Grandma states, "Come on, eat, enjoy!"

"I really shouldn't," the twins protest.

Their grandmother's face begins to take on that familiar wounded look. They know the message those elderly eyes are conveying: Food is my way of showing you love. If you reject my food, you're rejecting my love. You wouldn't be that cruel, would you?

Reaction

Nancy	Carol
Chronic Dieter	*Instinctive Eater*
"Grandma," Nancy states, "you're great to remember my favorite dessert! Okay, cut me a really big piece!" (An hour later, Grandma is heard warning Nancy, "Unless you do something about your weight, you'll never get married!")	"Grandma, I love you," Carol laughs, "but there's no way that dessert is going to fit into this body! Wrap some up and I'll take it home with me when I leave. And please, not another word about food. You've fed me too well already."

Scene VII

Lunch with Co-Workers

It's noon and the twins are sitting at their office desks. Pam walks up to them. "Lunchtime!" she announces. "Come on. Jean and I are going to the deli."

Nancy and Carol reply that they're really not hungry and think they'll take a raincheck.

"Are you nuts?!" responds an incredulous Pam. "This company only gives one lunch break—noon to one. If you don't eat now, you'll have to wait till five! Your blood sugar will drop—you'll be starving. Come on!"

Reaction

Nancy *Chronic Dieter*	Carol *Instinctive Eater*
"You're right," Nancy says. "I'm going to be ravenous later. I'd better eat lunch now while I have the chance."	Carol replies, "I just can't eat preventively. I'm not hungry right now, and if I'm not hungry, I really don't want to eat. But thanks. I'll walk over to the deli with you and buy some fruit and rice cakes to keep in my desk, in case I get hungry later."

Scene VIII

The Family Dinner

It's 6:00 P.M. and the family—mother, father, brother, and sisters—are all seated at the dinner table. Nancy and Carol remark that they really don't feel hungry now.

"Well, it's dinner time and the family is eating," their mother answers. "We expect you to join us."

Reaction

Nancy *Chronic Dieter*	Carol *Instinctive Eater*
"Okay, Mom, fill up a plate for me," Nancy says.	"That's exactly what I intend to do," Carol says. "I'm going to just sit here with you, have a little something to drink and maybe a few bites of salad." When her mother asks if she'll feel deprived watching the others eat, Carol replies, "I'd feel deprived if I were hungry, but I'm not, so I won't. And I'm not left out, Mom. I don't need to eat to be with you."

Scene IX

Lunchtime at a Business Meeting

It's 1:30 in the afternoon and the twins are sitting around a conference table with the other execs—all male. The meeting has been going on since 11:30 this morning and there's still no end in sight. Nancy's and Carol's stomachs are gurgling; they're aware that for the last 10 minutes they've paid little attention to the topic of profit margins. All they've thought about is food.

Reaction

Nancy	Carol
Chronic Dieter	*Instinctive Eater*
Nancy waits until the meeting breaks up at 2:45. Barely able to contain herself, Nancy rushes to the nearest food source—the vending machine. By 2:52, she has scarfed down two cupcakes, one Milky Way, and a bag of potato chips.	Carol immediately pushes her chair back and says, "Gentlemen, let's take ten for a restroom break." As they exit, she heads to her desk (or her purse), where she reaches for her stash of rice cakes and an apple.

Conquering Bingeing: Why You've Always Failed

You now know from previous chapters that dieting triggers out-of-control bingeing and that the binges soon acquire lives of their own. (The habit of bingeing is another choice from which dieters have abdicated responsibility.) Overeaters binge for one major reason: *They don't have a good enough reason not to binge.* Of course, you can easily come up with a pack of good reasons to avoid bingeing. In fact, if you were to write them down, they might look something like this:

- I want to be thinner.
- I want to look and feel better.
- I want to be healthy.
- I want to set a good example for my children.
- I want to be around to watch my children grow up.
- I want to feel in control.

• I want to feel more comfortable in social situations.
• I want to feel more sexually uninhibited.
• I want others to admire my appearance.

They look great on paper, don't they? But in the context of your real life, they add up to this: *"I still binge!"*

Why? Unfortunately, when you're ensnared in the Diet Mentality, what's most important in your life—more important than your health, your wealth, or the well-being of your children—is your right to binge whenever you want to!

Yes, it's painful and a bit embarrassing to admit, but every time you eat out of control, your actions are proving that nothing takes priority over your right to binge.

Desire Is Not Motivation

Motivation can be defined as a measure of how moved you are to act. Paradoxically, as you've already learned, the obsessive need to be thinner is precisely what robs you of the necessary motivation to eat in control.

To prove that your desire to be thin will not motivate you to eat in control, think about certain situations that could occur in your life. For example, you're following a diet (begun when you still believed diets worked), and then your child becomes ill. Will your actions show that you are moved toward thinness (continuing with the diet) or that you're moved toward instant gratification (soothing your anxiety with food)?

Or suppose that, to fit into that gorgeous designer dress you want to wear to your daughter's upcoming wedding, you've been watching what you eat. But then, unexpectedly, you're fired from your job. Will your actions move you toward fitting into the dress or toward the refrigerator?

Or, you've recently started an exercise program, but then the IRS tells you that you must come up with $30,000 in back taxes. The only way you'll be able to pull this off is by selling your house. Will your actions move you toward the gym or toward instant gratification in the kitchen?

If you're a typical Overeater, no matter how passionately you *want* to be thinner, in times of stress or intense emotion, your motivation to binge will always be far stronger than your motivation to become thin. There is no such thing as having *enough* motivation to become thin—for anyone!

The First Secret of Self-Motivation: Self-Nurturance

Instinctive Eaters motivate themselves by remembering and acknowledging the answers to these two questions:

What is best for me? What nurtures me? They are aware that motivation is derivative of a larger concept: *Feeling good about themselves!*

An Instinctive Eater is also aware that it's neither nurturing nor "best" to dislike yourself, to judge yourself as unattractive, to consider yourself blameworthy or fault-ridden, to obsess about your weight, to weigh yourself (or let others weigh you), to own clothes that no longer fit, to hand over your personal power and allow others to vote on you, to tolerate applause or boos based on your weight loss, to neglect exercise, to diet, to deprive yourself of foods you enjoy, to eat junk food excessively, to do without nutritious food.

Instinctive Eaters almost always choose *not* to engage in these practices. Rather than consider themselves fat and ugly and inadequate, they consider themselves round and beautiful and terrific, and that helps to motivate them.

Interestingly, they know that they can go either way at any time. But, since both choices are arbitrary, they figure, "Why not choose the one that feels good?" (In the end, we each make it all up for ourselves, anyway.)

In the two following scenes, notice the vast difference between the self-nurturing focus of the two women. Carol takes care of her own needs by eating the foods she enjoys and by refusing to be caught in the Diet Mentality weight game.

Scene X

Dinner with Friends

Nancy and Carol have just finished eating dinner with six friends when the waiter appears wheeling the dessert cart. A freshly baked chocolate cheesecake immediately catches their eye. "I'm already full, I'd better pass this one up," they both think. But everyone at the crowded table is singing the praises of the cheesecake and they've all decided to order it.

Reaction

Nancy	Carol
Chronic Dieter	*Instinctive Eater*

Nancy — Chronic Dieter

"Well, I know I shouldn't, but if everyone else is, I can't resist," she says, then thinks to herself: "Besides, I don't want to be the odd man out." Now she begins berating herself: "That's so typical of you! What a glutton you are. Well, you'll pay for it in the morning when your stomach is all bloated out." Suddenly, Nancy looks at her plate and realizes it's empty. She was so busy castigating herself that even though she ate the cheesecake, she never really *tasted* it.

Carol — Instinctive Eater

"Well, friends," Carol says, "It looks good and I know it's going to taste good, so let's go for it! A little recreational eating never hurt anyone." Carol eats and enjoys every last bite. She doesn't have a single regret, nor does she give a single thought to her weight. In full control, she chose to give herself the pleasure of the delicious dessert, even though her body wasn't hungry. (Instinctive Eaters know that occasional recreational eating won't cause weight gain.)

Scene XI

At the Health Club

Having recently joined a health club to increase muscle tone, flexibility, and aerobic capacity, Nancy and Carol are talking to the instructor, who is filling in their goals on their program cards. Catching the twins off guard, she asks, "How much weight do you want to lose?"

Reaction

Nancy	Carol
Chronic Dieter	*Instinctive Dieter*

Nancy — Chronic Dieter

"I must be out of it," she thinks. "I guess getting in shape means losing weight. Well, maybe that's why I really came here, after all." To the instructor, she says, "You can write down 20 pounds."

Carol — Instinctive Dieter

"I didn't come here to lose weight," Carol replies. But the instructor persists, so Carol answers, "I'm not really concerned with weight." Flustered, the instructor blurts out that everyone wants to lose weight and asks again what to put on the card. "Put whatever you want," Carol impatiently responds, "but let's get on with the program."

The Result of Self-Motivation by Self-Nurturance

When you choose to believe that you're fine (if not perfect) just the way you are, you'll begin to enjoy incredible freedom. And when you decide to commit your life to nurturing yourself by respecting yourself, the desire to binge becomes less compelling. Your focus changes. You gain virtually effortless control around food. The following situations should help you out.

Scene XII

Avoiding the Binge before Dinner

It's 4:00 on a Saturday afternoon. Nancy and Carol have just finished shopping and are beginning to feel hungry.

Reaction

Nancy	**Carol**
Chronic Dieter	*Instinctive Eater*
"I'd better resist this hunger," she says to herself. "Dinner is at 6:00 and if I eat now, I'll spoil my appetite. It's just a matter of willpower. If I really care about my weight, I won't eat. But look at those cookies in that bakery window! I just can't! Hang in there, kid!" After obsessing for ½ hour, Nancy finds herself back at the bakery, this time eating cookies from a large bag. Ten minutes later, she's sighing to herself, "I can't believe I ate the entire dozen!"	"Dinner is at 6:00, and I really don't want to spoil my appetite," Carol thinks. "I'll just have a few bites of fruit or a bran muffin to take the edge off my hunger."

Scene XIII

Avoiding the Binge at the Supermarket

It's 1:00 on Saturday afternoon and the twins need to do some grocery shopping. They enter the supermarket.

Reaction

| **Nancy** | **Carol** |
| *Chronic Dieter* | *Instinctive Eater* |

Nancy hasn't eaten lunch and she is starving! On impulse, she dives for the items she's moved toward when she gets too hungry. Her cart fills up with cakes, ice cream, pastries, candies, sodas, TV dinners, canned foods with sugary syrups, processed cheeses, chips, pretzels, and sugar-loaded cereals. She's ready for a binge.

Carol pulls out her shopping list. She has eaten before shopping, so she won't be tempted to buy impulsively. Her list includes nutritious foods that she enjoys and a couple of maybe-not-so-nutritious items that she likes, wants, and intends to treat herself to later.

The Secret of Focusing on Your Needs

The obsession with thinness is not a simple quirk. For Chronic Dieters, it becomes a smoke screen that conceals their real needs. Instead of focusing on who you are, what you need, and what you want to be doing with your life, gratification in these areas is delayed. You hold on to that same magical thought: Thinness resolves all conflicts.

When the pursuit of thinness stops and the pursuit of self-nurturance begins, you begin to meet your real needs appropriately. You take your life off hold, and no longer wait for that moment when you've lost those 4 (or 40) pounds.

As you'll see below, keeping yourself on the back burner until you feel thin and attractive affects every aspect of your life.

Scene XIV

Personal Tasks

At 7:00 in the evening, Nancy and Carol arrive home from a long, weary workday. A stack of ironing piled on the back of a chair reminds them that the 11th hour has arrived. If the ironing isn't done tonight, tomorrow they may be forced to wear whatever's left in the closet.

Standing in front of the ironing board, they bicker over whose turn it is to do the hateful chore. Disgruntled, edgy, and tired, they decide that this particular task is not only a real drag, but a drain. There's no doubt about it—it's time for a break.

Reaction

Nancy
Chronic Dieter
She heads into the kitchen and takes a ½-hour "snack" break.

Carol
Instinctive Eater
She heads for the kitchen, then stops herself. "Wait a minute!" she says out loud. "I'm not hungry—I'm tired!" She walks into the bedroom, lies down for a while, then, feeling refreshed, returns to the ironing. She finishes the task in half her usual time, with no sweat.

Scene XV

Buying Clothes

The twins have just received a catalog of the new spring line from a department store. As they flip through the pages, they each spot a dress, a skirt, and a pair of leather pants that really appeal to them. Both realize that it's been quite some time since they treated themselves to beautiful new clothes, and both really need to augment their wardrobes.

Reaction

Nancy
Chronic Dieter
She tells herself that tomorrow she's heading right down to that store—well, maybe not tomorrow. But as soon as she loses 20 pounds. (Somehow, the new clothes are never purchased.)

Carol
Instinctive Eater
She tells herself that tomorrow she's heading right down to that store—and does. She buys the dress, the skirt, and the leather pants (in the size that fits her comfortably), wears them immediately, and feels gorgeous.

The Ultimate Secret

There are days when you feel motivated and actually get the job done, even though it's unpleasant. There are other days when you don't feel motivated and nothing gets done. The difference in your response on those two days can be attributed to how you use your mind. What is the secret mindset of Instinctive Eaters? How do they motivate themselves? Listen carefully.

Last week, you anticipated an unpleasant task—maybe that aerobics class where you grunt, groan, sweat, suffer sore muscles, and have trouble catching your breath. What a bummer! You decided to skip it. But why?

In your mind, you pictured yourself straining; you heard yourself grunting and groaning; you felt your sticky sweat; you experienced your heavy breathing and sore muscles.

This week, however, you went to the class. Now why?

This time you pictured your future. You saw your taut body effortlessly walking miles, climbing stairs, and keeping up with your kids; you heard your self-congratulations at the end of the class for a job well done; you felt your increased energy level; you experienced your sense of accomplishment and your pride in honoring your commitment; and you reveled in the well-deserved, hot, soothing shower on your skin.

Do you see the difference? When your mind focuses on the *impending* task, you lose motivation. But when your mind focuses on the *completed* task—when it jumps to the future—you gain motivation.

The simple but powerful secret of self-motivation is to focus not on the effort but on the result of that effort. Try to form compelling visual images of your desired result. Hear your inner voice proffering great amounts of approval for completing the task. Feel the relief, the joy, the pride—every powerful emotion—you'll experience upon completion.

If these images, messages, and feelings are strong enough, you'll never have to worry about being out of control or lacking motivation. Once you have begun to visualize the enormous self-satisfaction to be gained from completing the task, you'll have found the first key to the self-motivation you've been seeking.

Scene XVI

Exercise Class

This time the twins are in their gym, nearly finished with their workouts. They're both tired, a little short of breath, sweaty, bored, and on the edge of quitting. After all, they reason, three-quarters of a workout is still a pretty good showing.

Reaction

Nancy *Chronic Dieter*	**Carol** *Instinctive Eater*
She visualizes another 15 minutes of sore muscles—and quits.	She visualizes how proud she's going to feel when she finishes her workout—and continues to the end.

The Internal Saboteur

"But I don't think I'll ever be able to use these secrets," you're probably thinking to yourself right about now. "Something tells me I just won't succeed." Don't worry about those thoughts. All human beings are equipped with what I call the Internal Saboteur, an inner voice that fights to control us. It's a powerful force, and one that must be acknowledged. But the more it wins, the less successful we are.

The Internal Saboteur is an automatic mechanism of the mind designed to protect us from perceived unpleasantness or shock. Since the Internal Saboteur can't reason, it doesn't discriminate: It employs a blanket method to ward off pain.

The goal of the Internal Saboteur is to prevent us from confronting new experiences by confining us to old, habitual behaviors. It neither recognizes nor understands that many of these habits are exactly what cause us pain. (It does know, however, that eating chocolate bars is less risky than voicing outrage at a spouse, a lover, a friend, or a boss.)

The Internal Saboteur responds to your good intentions with strong and forbidding visual images. As these images flash on your mental screen, you're provided with graphic details of the disaster in which all your plans will end. The Internal Saboteur's pictures of humiliation and failure are geared to ensure that you won't start the new business, wear sexy lingerie for your spouse, or even walk across the room to meet that interesting-looking stranger.

You already know the repetitive lyrics to the Internal Saboteur's unrelenting song.

You can't do that . . . Go ahead and quit . . . It won't work . . . You don't deserve that . . . You're too fat . . . You'll be rejected . . . You'll never amount to anything . . . It's wrong to feel bad—stuff that emotion! . . . Don't set goals—you'll never reach them . . . You're not good enough. . . .

The Internal Saboteur can begin to sing its siren song anywhere, at any time, and for the most foolish of reasons. Consider this scene.

Scene XVII

Comparing Yourself to Others

Nancy and Carol are in the locker room changing before their workout when they spot a tall, thin, "gorgeous" woman.

Reaction

Nancy	Carol
Chronic Dieter	*Instinctive Eater*
She feels instant animosity. Her Internal Saboteur tells her there is no point in starting a conversation—this woman is obviously stuck-up and feels far too superior to talk to someone as fat as Nancy.	She hears the Internal Saboteur, but ignores it and strikes up an interesting conversation about the tough class this hour. She chooses not to be threatened by this stranger's beauty.

Scene XVIII

Diet Books

Nancy and Carol are browsing through a bookstore when they see a stunning photograph of a slim Elizabeth Taylor on the cover of her diet book. They begin to think about diets and how they've never been successful following one.

Reaction

Nancy	Carol
Chronic Dieter	*Instinctive Eater*
"But look what this one did for Liz!" her Internal Saboteur tells her. "Maybe *this* is the one. Besides, don't you owe it to yourself to try *something?*" Nancy responds by purchasing the book.	"This is a seductive cover," Carol thinks. Then she intercepts her Internal Saboteur by saying to herself, "But why should I believe that a book written by a noncredentialed person who happens to be a superstar would be the answer?" Carol passes up the book, and a few years later, spotting pictures of the author looking nothing like that slim cover photo, feels a sense of justification.

The Secret of Conquering the Internal Saboteur

Sorry. None of us can totally conquer the Internal Saboteur. As you saw in the above scenes, even Instinctive Eaters tussle with it. It never goes away—it never dies. But if you remember this one thought, your life will never be the same: *What your Internal Saboteur tells you doesn't matter!*

All of us—Chronic Dieters *and* Instinctive Eaters—are stuck with the Internal Saboteur. We see the same disastrous images, hear the same lyric line. But again, we respond differently. When new Instinctive Eaters hear the Internal Saboteur, they simply disregard its message. After years of being habitually ignored, this meddling singer's transmission signal becomes extremely weak. Instinctive Eaters realize its voice is still there, but it's a faint, ever fainter voice.

On the other hand, as a Chronic Dieter, you hear the Internal Saboteur and you take its message seriously! You believe it's sending useful, important information that should be acted upon! Worse, you often delude yourself into thinking that by dieting to thinness, its paralyzing images and messages will cease and you'll then be able to begin your life!

Not so. Instinctive Eaters know that thinness will neither obliterate nor intimidate the Internal Saboteur. They've learned that by refusing to give credence to its messages, they conserve enormous amounts of energy. They are keenly aware that the "intelligence" they receive from the Internal Saboteur is contrary to how they want to *feel* and what they want to *do.*

There's only one way to live the life you often fantasize—ignore the Internal Saboteur.

As one seminar participant remarked, "It's such a relief to know that I don't have to change its messages. It seems so much easier to just hear them and refuse to act on them."

Scene XIX

Surrounded by Dieters

Sitting around the lounge during lunch, a group of women flip through a stack of women's magazines, discussing the latest diet. As Nancy and Carol (who have now sworn off diets) enter the room, their colleagues begin expressing their excitement and asking if the twins think this diet will work.

Reaction

Nancy
Chronic Dieter

"See what they have to say," her Internal Saboteur advises. "You don't want to appear unfriendly!" Nancy is quickly sucked into the conversation about dieting.

Carol
Instinctive Eater

Carol is slightly intrigued, but realizes it is the Internal Saboteur at work. She remembers this is an old habit. "I wouldn't know if it works," she says, smiling pleasantly, "I don't diet anymore." When her friend Pam insists that Carol knows a lot about diets and presses her for an opinion, Carol says, "I just don't know, Pam. I stopped dieting." The women shrug and slowly turn their attention away from Carol, who then continues about her business.

The Secret of Negative Emotional Responses

Contrary to popular opinion, emotions provide us with very little informational value. For example, although guilt informs us that we have violated our ethical standards, anxiety informs us that we should be prepared, and fear informs us that we must protect ourselves, the information this triumvirate provides for us is primitive. Our intelligent, analytical, evolved human minds actually provide us with much more useful information.

Emotions are transient. One emotion possesses us, lingers for a while, and then is replaced by another. The process repeats itself endlessly. Whether we consciously do or do not want a particular emotion isn't relevant. An emotion will march in uninvited in response to something very big or nothing very much, and, just as unexpectedly, depart.

What informational value do these transitory emotions offer us? More to the point, what are we supposed to *do* with them? According to common theory, we're supposed to "control" them, but the health consequences of controlling emotions are nothing less than disastrous.

In our society, it's still taboo to allow ourselves to experience so-called negative emotions—anxiety, worry, guilt, or fear; boredom, sadness, loneliness, or depression. We feel compelled to control them, or in the vernacular, to stuff them down. The question lingers: If emotions are transitory and undependable, and if our attempts at suppression are ultimately damaging, again, what is their purpose?

They have only one purpose: *to be experienced.* (In fact, I sometimes tell my seminar participants that emotions have the same significance as bowel movements—they only become important when we *stop* experiencing them.)

Chronic Dieters believe that every negative emotion is a call to eat, to rid themselves of the unpleasant intruder by stuffing it down with ice cream or doughnuts. Instinctive Eaters would never think of pairing sadness with pizza, anxiety with potato chips, or boredom with chocolate. They've learned to disassociate food from emotions and to go for the nurturing that's needed. When they're hurt, angry, or depressed, they move toward the noneating solution that fits the emotion.

Scene XX

Family Crisis

Nancy and Carol are in the hospital listening to some extremely troublesome news concerning their mother's health. "I'm sorry," the doctor tells them, "I know your mother's been here for two weeks, but her heart attack was severe and I can't make any predictions about her prognosis."

The twins leave the hospital in a daze—anxious and distraught, feeling helpless, panicky, and alone. When they arrive home, they look for a way to soothe themselves. Without realizing it, before their coats are off, they're peering into the refrigerator.

Reaction

Nancy	Carol
Chronic Dieter	*Instinctive Eater*
She transfers the contents of the refrigerator into her stomach and then manages to take off her coat. Ten minutes later, Nancy feels	"Slow down, Carol," she tells herself. "Take a big, deep breath. There's nothing in this refrigerator that's going to solve your wor-

Nancy	Carol
stuffed and guilty—and she is still worried sick about her mother's condition.	ries about Mom. What you need is some support." Carol takes off her coat and calls a close friend.

The Secret of Reaching Your Goals: Commitment

You can't depend on your emotions to support you in reaching your goals—zipping in and out as they do, they're just too undependable. (In fact, most people who *do* reach their goals do so *in spite of* their emotions!) But, just as you must be willing to listen to the nasty repetitive lyrics of the Internal Saboteur without acting on them, you must be willing to simply *experience* your negative emotions—to just *have* them—without acting on them.

Difficult to pull off? Yes. However, there is one tool powerful enough to resist the combined enemy forces of our negative emotions and our Internal Saboteur: our commitment.

Scene XXI

Exercise Class

The twins have arrived home from work tonight feeling somewhat tired. "I don't feel like going to my exercise class," each thinks to herself. "It's pouring out. My leotard needs to be washed. I'm tired. Skipping one class won't hurt. I'm just not in the mood."

Reaction

Nancy	Carol
Chronic Dieter	*Instinctive Eater*
Controlled by her emotions and her Internal Saboteur, Nancy stays home.	Guided by her commitment, Carol goes to class.

The Diet Mentality Response to Commitment

As a Chronic Dieter, you often lose the capacity to distinguish between a commitment and a short-lived New Year's resolution. You've broken your commitments to yourself so many times, you've lost faith in your own promises.

There's little to wonder about. Through your history of broken promises to all those diets with their built-in failure guarantees, you've lost faith in your own word. You've continually promised to achieve the unachievable—to lower your weight permanently through dieting. Of course you have no trust in your commitments! By believing the lie that diets work, you've created an inner atmosphere of self-suspicion and mistrust. As a victim of the Diet Mentality, you've forgotten that commitments *do* work. More important, you don't know how to experience a lapse without feeling that you've totally blown the commitment.

The Secret of Making Commitments That Work

I define a commitment as "a 100 percent go-for." A commitment defines your operating framework. This means that within the framework of your commitment, you will put forth your 100 percent best effort. As a Chronic Dieter, you confuse "100 percent go-for" with "all-or-nothing," "do-it-perfectly," "don't-blow-the-diet" thinking. You believe that once you participate in a "wrong" act, you've blown it. Face it, you've come to equate commitments with diets.

True commitments can't be blown. They are an operating framework that defines an area of your life to which you must always return.

Scene XXII

Caring for Yourself

A while back, in an unusual coincidence, each of the twins severely sprained an ankle and was laid up for some time, unable to move. As a result of their inactivity and overeating, they now notice that their clothes are too tight.

Reaction

Nancy *Chronic Dieter*	Carol *Instinctive Eater*
She runs to the scale to check out her "score" and sees a weight gain	She doesn't own a scale, wouldn't use it if she did, and wouldn't

Nancy	**Carol**
of several pounds. Shocked, upset, and panicky, she vows to go on a diet immediately.	think of letting a number determine her state of mind. She knows she's been inactive, eating too much, and snacking on the wrong foods. Her mirror and clothes confirm what she already knows. She vows to return to her healthy eating habits and activities, knowing her weight gain will take care of itself soon enough.

The Secret of Sticking to Your Commitment

As I stated earlier, you eat out of control because your reasons for giving up bingeing aren't good enough. The only reason that would be compelling enough to make you respond to food as an Instinctive Eater would be a commitment to self-nurturance—to your own health and well-being.

If you commit to do your 100 percent best to control bingeing, here's my guarantee: You will fall flat on your face over and over again.

And that's fine! You're a beginning Instinctive Eater, and beginners are expected to fall down. Remember, for years you've been habitually eating emotionally. Now you're introducing a new, alien habit to your system—eating in response to your Body Signals. You're human; that means your 100 percent best will be less than perfect.

If you live your life in the framework of your commitment, you won't have blown it if you binge. You will merely have failed to act consistently with your commitment. Again, remember—this is not a diet! Your only job is to notice, to learn something about yourself from the lapse, and then to return to your commitment *without judgment.*

This is not an excuse to break your commitment flagrantly. It's a chance for you to observe and learn more about how it's reinforced. Every time you break your commitment but return to it, your commitment is strengthened. Like certain tests we took in school, there are no points taken off for wrong answers: Only right answers count.

Each time you feel it's binge time and you find a more self-nurturing alternative behavior, you reinforce and strengthen your transition to instinctive eating.

Scene XXIII

When Life Turns Upside Down

Life hasn't been going well for Nancy and Carol. Their lovers have left them. Massive layoffs at work are jeopardizing their jobs. The twins have been eating out of control and gaining weight, and now feel totally depressed. Looking in the mirror, they feel even worse: like fat, bloated, ugly slobs.

Reaction

Nancy	Carol
Chronic Dieter	*Instinctive Eater*
Nancy feels hopeless and defeated. She continues to rationalize her bingeing by telling herself: "I've already gained the weight anyway, and life is so bad that I deserve to soothe myself the quick and easy way—with food."	"I'm deeply into the Woman's Model," she tells herself. "I have not blown anything; this is a state of 'breakdown'—a temporary condition in which I've broken my commitment to myself. I know what to do. Acknowledge it. Recommit to my original goals. Get some support!" Carol calls a close, encouraging friend to help her through this very bad time.

The Secret of Creating the Instinctive Eater's Reality

You're now totally familiar with the reality of the Internal Saboteur. It tells you what's wrong with you (you're too fat!), what to do about it (diet!), and how to feel (unacceptable and/or out of control). The messages of the Internal Saboteur emerge effortlessly.

To become an Instinctive Eater, it's now time to create a new set of messages. Take a look at the following list. Yes, at first they'll feel stilted and unnatural, and it may require a bit of an effort for you to repeat them. But after some practice, they'll begin to feel familiar, "right," and slowly take the place of the old lies you've told yourself. Stop here for a moment and try them out.

"Today I choose that no one gets to vote on my body or my eating habits."

"Today I choose that nurturing myself is my most important project."

"Today I choose to experience all of my emotions and be guided by my commitments."

"Today I choose that I'm fine the way I am—that I'm a terrific person."

"Today I choose that thinness is beautiful, but *my* looks are equally beautiful."

"Today I choose to believe all these things."

"Today I choose to feel all these things."

Learn—Do—Feel

I've heard all your objections to these new messages many times over. "They're fine for other people," you say, "but I don't believe them for myself." Since you really don't "feel" them, you think it's pointless to give them credence by repeating them to yourself.

At this point, having been an eyewitness to the differences in the responses of Nancy and Carol, it should be clear that unless you *do* believe and feel these messages, you'll repeatedly wind up thinking, feeling, and behaving like Nancy. There's no doubt about what her entire life will look like. When she finally leaves this Earth, the epitaph on her tombstone will probably read: She only had 10 pounds to go.

The mistake that victims of the Diet Mentality make is in believing that actions result from feelings. As Nancy might say, "When I feel more comfortable about my appearance, then I'll put on a bathing suit and enjoy the beach."

Don't hold your breath waiting.

For Nancy to feel comfortable in a bathing suit, she must take some *active* steps. She'll have to begin by telling herself:

All these years, I've let my Internal Saboteur tell me I'm too fat and I've bought into it. I've listened to my well-meaning and not-so-well-meaning friends and family tell me I'm too fat and I've bought into it. I've let the media tell me I'm too fat and I've bought into it. All my 'buying in' has brought me nothing but misery. I'm

tired of listening to my Internal Saboteur (and to my external sab-
oteurs as well!). I deserve to feel great and have it all in this body,
the body I'm in right now—today.

Then Nancy must act. Even though she'll feel shaky in her new resolve,
she must put on the bathing suit and go to the beach, or buy the great
outfit and go to the class reunion. The more she acts, the more her
feelings of fear, embarrassment, and discomfort will be replaced by feelings of confidence, comfort, and entitlement.

If Nancy feels she's fat and ugly, the world will agree. If Nancy
feels she's beautiful and terrific, the world will agree. The choice is in
her hands.

From Overeater
to Instinctive Eater

Becoming an Instinctive Eater means that you are now clear that you
are in control of food and therefore, weight. (In chapter 9, you'll learn
how to tune in to your Body Signals and handle sweet cravings.)

For now, though, you must begin to think like someone who is in
control of food. That means you:

- Do not allow anyone else to vote on your appearance.
- Create the "true" reality for yourself and give up the "lie."
- Say no and yes to your own mealtimes and stay faithful to your own
  Body Signals.
- Motivate yourself to change because you care about yourself (*not* be-
  cause your defective, fat body should be a perfect, thin one).
- Divorce yourself from the Diet Mentality in conversations with
  others.
- Focus on your true needs, stop concealing them with binges, and stop
  imagining that future thinness will take care of them.
- Keep yourself motivated by focusing on your end results.
- Ignore your Internal Saboteur.
- Have the courage to experience your emotions.
- Disassociate your emotions from your commitments.
- Don't "undo" overeating by dieting.
- Avoid the seduction of the diet industry propaganda.
- Stay alert and conscious of your commitments for dealing with food.

The Final Result

You now know the secrets of Instinctive Eaters. You know how they think, feel, and behave. If you make their secrets a deliberate part of your daily consciousness, you will be *doing* what Instinctive Eaters *do*. You will love yourself, and out of loving yourself, you will love your body. Out of loving your body, you will respond to your Body Signals— feed your body when it's hungry and stop when it's satisfied. This means you will nurture it by feeding it whenever it wants, whatever it wants, as much as it wants—in total control and at peace.

You're about to be welcomed into the fold of the 4½ billion people who maintain a stable weight!

Chapter 6

Accepting Your Body— Loving It!

Acceptance is an act of self-love.
A person who responds to her
Body Signals is a person who loves
herself and accepts her body.

Before you can become comfortable as a member of the 4½ billion people who respond to their Body Signals and instinctively maintain a stable weight, there are still a few steps to go.

But first, I'd like you to listen in on a conversation between me and a Chronic Dieter named Gloria who volunteered to be questioned in front of the group at a recent seminar.

Dialogue with a Dieter

Steve: Gloria, are you fat?

Gloria: I feel as if I am.

Steve: How fat are you?

Gloria: I could stand to lose 14 pounds.

Steve: Okay. If you were 14 pounds less than your current weight, you'd be at your ideal weight. How long have you been above that ideal weight?

Gloria: On and off for about eight years.

Steve: Out of the last eight years, what percentage of time would you estimate you were at your ideal weight?

Gloria: Ten percent of the time.

Steve: So, you've been fat 90 percent of the last eight years?

Gloria: Not exactly. First of all, this is the heaviest I've been—I haven't always been at this weight. Secondly, it's not that I'm really *fat!* I'm heavy, I guess.

Steve: Fourteen pounds *less* is "thin" and right now you're "heavy." At what weight does "heavy" begin?

Gloria: I never thought about it like that. I'd say 11 or 12 pounds up.

Steve: Then what would you call 10 pounds up?

Gloria: I call that plump.

Steve: Where does "plump" begin?

Gloria: Six pounds up.

Steve: Then what do you call 5 pounds up?

Gloria: Overweight.

Steve: You say you're "heavy," not "fat." How much weight do you have to gain to pass from "heavy" to "fat"?

Gloria: I think if I were 20 pounds above my ideal weight, then I'd be fat.

Steve: I want to make sure that I'm following you. At 14 pounds less, you're "thin." Add 5 pounds and you're "overweight." At 10 or 11 pounds up, you're "plump." From 12 to 19 pounds up, you're "heavy," and at 20 pounds, you're "fat."

Gloria: I feel as if I'm sounding silly.

Steve: That's not my intention. My intention is for you to realize how tyrannized you are by numbers. You assign significance to numbers that are in reality, arbitrary and meaningless, then suffer from the meaning you attach to them. Given the culture you live in, I wouldn't use the word "silly." I'd use words like "sad, understandable, self-defeating, self-degrading, self-crippling." Do you believe the numbers game has crippled you?

Gloria: Yes, in many ways. When I don't weigh what I should, I don't feel good about myself.

Steve: And can you explain how that costs you?

For the sake of brevity, my questions have been edited out of Gloria's explanation, which follows.

Gloria's Explanation

"I'm in real estate," she began. "When I feel good about my appearance, I'm very confident around my clients. When I feel fat, I'm distracted. I really enjoy my work and don't believe I've ever lost a sale because of how I feel, but when I feel too heavy, I'm so aware of it that my enjoyment is drained out. I feel like I have to work three times as hard with my clients to make the sale.

"Before I got married," she continued, "I turned down dates solely because I felt too ugly. Because of how I felt about my appearance, I missed a lot of parties and outings to the beach. I was either too depressed to go or too unwilling to deal with the fear of what I imagined people must be thinking of me.

"I also know my sex life isn't what it could be," she added. "It was much better when I was thinner. Now I avoid sex much more often. I don't like my husband seeing me naked when the lights are on—I get distracted wondering how he can enjoy making love to someone with all this excess flesh. The funny thing is, he tells me he thinks I'm perfect! The fool!" she laughed, "What does he know?"

At this point, I said to Gloria, "For 90 percent of the last eight years, you've been above your ideal weight." She nodded. "This may be a strange proposition," I continued, "but try to get a handle on the time you spend experiencing your feelings as opposed to the time you spend active and busy. Because of your feelings about your weight, what percentage of those feelings do you estimate are painful?"

She answered: "At least 50 percent."

During this dialogue (which is replayed again and again at every seminar), the other participants look on with a mixture of horror, fear, and loathing. They have good reason. You see, *Gloria is 5 feet, 7 inches tall and weighs 129 pounds.*

What's *She* Got to Gripe About?

Gloria's answers and explanations reverberate in the other participants' minds. Yes, she expresses their feelings and uses their words, but no—her message doesn't compute! "When you look like her, you're supposed to feel differently," one woman explained. "Those feelings are only justifiable if you're *my* size!" stated another, "She has no reason to feel like that!" "After all," a third woman noted, "she has a body I'd kill to have!"

Still, the group's emotions are mixed. They can't get a grip on their feelings about Gloria. On the one hand, they're appalled that she is so tyrannized by—and nonaccepting of—her body. On the other hand, they empathize completely. These women live with those same feelings every day of their lives and don't believe it's fair to invalidate her experience. Caught between a rock and a hard place, the other Chronic Dieters have to admit:

Thinness does not guarantee happiness. The proof is standing in front of them. They begin to understand that size is immaterial; it's the perception that counts—and the terrible feelings that accompany that perception.

They're right. These women are no more justified in the nonacceptance of their bodies at their weight than Gloria is of her body at her weight. They should be no more appalled by her numbers obsession, her distraction with clients, her unwillingness to go on dates and to parties, her avoidance of sex, and her need to belittle her husband's compliments than they are by their own fears, self-flagellation, and body loathing. Gloria's fellow participants are *equally nonaccepting of their bodies.*

The "Dream Girl"

Given her height, her weight, and her "gorgeous looks," (in the eyes of other women), Gloria represents the female dream. Yet, she feels she's caught in a nightmare. Just ask her. She'll willingly tell you exactly which parts of her body are flawed and why she won't be at peace until they're fixed.

Gloria isn't alone. A famous talk show hostess recently did a show on women who hate parts of their bodies (as if there were women who didn't!). The show opened with a panel of models dressed in leotards who pointed out their flawed body parts—"My breasts are too large." "My legs are too thick." "My torso is too short." The audience responded to them with the same disbelief, disdain, and empathy as the seminar participants did to Gloria.

There's a not-so-funny joke I like to tell in my seminars. It goes like this. What's the major difference between men and women? Men have *bodies* and women have *body parts*. ("It's my hips—they bulge!" "It's my stomach—I hate it!" "It's my arms—they are just gross!" "It's my backside—it embarrasses me!") So it would seem that while men's bodies are made by God, women's body parts are made by Frank Perdue.

The obsession with thinness is rampant. And so is the myth that your feelings will change, your experience will change, your life will change when your least favorite body part is altered, when your body is small, when the number on the scale is lower. (Look at Gloria!) To women, weight and warfare have become synonymous.

The battle between you and your body, however, is about to come to an end.

You only have to do one thing: *Totally accept your body exactly as it is now.*

Acceptance: What It Is

Stick with me. Before you throw your hands up, listen to what acceptance means and what it can do for you.

Acceptance means that anything that you would do or feel if you had your ideal body, you will do or feel in this body.

If you would feel beautiful in a smaller body, then acceptance means you will feel beautiful in this one.

If you would feel confident with a differently shaped body part, then acceptance means you'll feel confident with the body part that belongs to you now.

If you would feel at peace with a thinner body, then acceptance means you'll feel at peace with the body you're in.

Acceptance means that you define the perfect body as the body you have today!

Acceptance: What It Isn't

It isn't resignation.

Acceptance doesn't mean resigning yourself to your fate as an unfortunate, overweight person.

Let me explain. In one of my seminars, a woman named Sherry listened to my definition of acceptance, then broke in. "I *do* accept my body," she vehemently stated. "I'm successful at my work. I have an active social life. I play tennis. I even make love with the lights on. I do everything with this body!"

On further questioning, Sherry backed down. She admitted that her protestations contained a subtle but profound lie. Sherry's accomplishments weren't achieved *with her body;* they were achieved *despite her body.* She perceived her size—emotionally and intellectually—as a handicap, more like a birthmark covering half of her face or a limb missing from her body. When she spoke, it was with the pride of a successful but genuinely handicapped person.

Acceptance does not mean grace under pressure or success in the face of adversity. Nor does acceptance mean making peace with your (perceived) handicap. Acceptance means seeing your body as *problem-free.*

When you accept your body, you are at peace with it and begin to feel genuinely "right" on the street, at the office, on the beach, in the bedroom, in groups, in the world.

Acceptance: Why?

If you don't accept your body completely, if you don't like or even love your body as it is now, you won't respond to your Body Signals and you won't achieve a permanently stable weight.

Why? For these two major reasons.

First: Nonacceptance is a disease that poisons your re-

sponses to your body. In your lust to change its size, you're driven to radical, unnatural actions—dieting, bulimia, exercise bulimia (exercise not to maintain fitness, but only to *eat more*), anorexia, and a variety of other torturous experiences. Nonacceptance is toxic: It produces feelings of anguish and despair that dominate your inner landscape. And let's face it—the drive to relieve those feelings is always greater than the need to nurture your body.

Acceptance *will* motivate you to care for your body. Let me tell you about Diane, one of my seminar graduates. After 35 years of dieting, she attended a seminar and then spent six months trying to tune into her Body Signals. During that time, she lost no weight. But soon after her period of adjustment, *without dieting,* her blouse size shrank from size 42 to 14. Had she been nonaccepting—lusting for rapid change and struggling to quell those terrible feelings of body loathing—Diane would have had neither the patience nor the perseverance to continue nurturing herself through all those months with no apparent result.

Until the birth of her son 35 years ago, Diane had been a size 4. Had she refused to accept her body, not only would she have continued to neglect her Body Signals, but she would also have found no peace with anything less than a return to size 4. Acceptance has provided her with both the impulse and the consciousness to nurture her body—to respond to its Hunger Signals and Satisfaction Signals—and to care for all of its needs.

Second: It's just basic common sense. Which do you take care of better, that which you dislike or that which you love and treasure?

Picture this: You're cleaning up the house and find yourself about to dust two objects on an end table. One, a clunky candlestick given to you by an office colleague, reflects neither your taste nor your standards. Basically, you dislike it. The other, given to you by your mother, is a delicate glass vase that reflects the family history and expresses your sense of aesthetics. Basically, you love it. The candlestick will probably receive a quick slapdash of the cloth, which may or may not topple it (you really don't care), while the vase will be handled with tenderness and regarded with affection (you really *do* care).

You don't have to reach to make the analogy work. As long as you refuse to accept your body, you'll treat it like the clunky, distasteful candlestick. But when you do accept your body, you'll treat it like the delicate, treasured vase. Look to your own experience: Can't you see that disliking your body moves you to abuse it?

Responding to your Body Signals isn't abuse—it's an act of self-love. It means that your body has value to you and must be given your tender attention. It's like a child. If you love your body the way you love your child, or would love your child if you had one, your body will return that love with strength, energy, and good feelings.

"Since I started thinking of my body as my child," Denise, a new Instinctive Eater, commented, "I'm less resistant to getting up and out to my aerobics class. Instead of saying, '*I* have to do this grueling chore,' I tell myself my *body* needs the workout, and if I neglect it, it's going to turn on me!" Like Denise, new Instinctive Eaters who have learned to respond to their Body Signals and are maintaining a stable weight now cherish their bodies as they would a child. You can see it: They exercise their bodies, feed their bodies nutritious foods, give their bodies pleasure, and receive pleasure back.

If you won't speak up for your body and accept it the way you would your child, who will? Until you regard your body as whole and worthy of your love, you'll continue to neglect and abuse it. Once you accept your body as a source of pleasure and pride, you'll be genuinely moved to pay attention to its needs, to respond to its signals, to nurture it with a new sense of reverence.

Acceptance: When?

Now.

Acceptance is not a process. It's a decision.

Helen, another seminar participant, offered the standard argument: "I've disliked my body for 40 years. There's no way I can just suddenly decide to like it!"

She's wrong. The length of time you've hated your body doesn't correlate with the length of time it takes to like it.

Liking your body is an instantaneous decision. It simply requires a firm declaration: "Enough is enough! Hating this body has only produced more pain and more pounds. If this is the body I have, so be it. I'm fine and I think it's beautiful!"

Will you be instantly comfortable with this new notion? Not necessarily. In that respect, Helen is right. It may take time. But, the declaration must be made immediately. The move to self-acceptance must start now. The perception of yourself as beautiful must begin today.

Acceptance: Who?

You . . .

. . . *no matter what you weigh.* The concept of acceptance is not only for thinner people—it's not an idea for you to adopt after you've lost more weight. To free yourself from the food-and-numbers tyranny, you must switch your self-perception! Until you can look at your body through a prism of acceptance and self-love, you'll continue to serve your scale and neglect your Body Signals! Acceptance will change your focus. Acceptance will allow you to experience a profound sense of peace exactly where you are right now (maybe for the first time in your life!). Most important: Acceptance will give you the freedom to act.

One note of caution: This is not an "Acceptance Diet." Your focus must be on accepting your body to experience a peace with it—to let you nurture it and let it nurture you. If you are currently above setpoint and your weight drops—you've won. You'll then begin the process of accepting a new, smaller body. If you've already lost all the weight you're going to lose—you've won. You will have achieved a new sense of self, a sense of dignity, and you will have found a profound sense of peace.

Acceptance: How?

Just do it.

Walk the walk of the "beautiful people." Buy the fashionable clothes. Wear the forbidden bathing suit. Go to the class reunion that's coming up. Make the appointment for the interview. Give the speech. Invite him over for a candlelight dinner. Accept the dates. Dance. Sing!

Start doing whatever makes you feel beautiful and part of the world. It will happen. You'll soon feel comfortable with and entitled to your new perceptions and your new life. You'll be amazed.

Summary: Your Objections

For victims of the Diet Mentality, acceptance is the most difficult concept to absorb. Even as you read, your Internal Saboteur is rejecting the idea of acceptance and planting a number of objections in your mind to obscure the truth.

Since you can't avoid the Internal Saboteur, let me state the ten objections you're raising and answer them for you.

Objection 1: "How can you tell me to like my appearance—much less *love* it—when I'm so fat?"

Answer: As a Chronic Dieter, it seems to you that the word "fat" has been removed from the dictionary and replaced by a far more descriptive phrase—*fat and ugly.* When stating this objection, here's what you really mean: "How can I accept my fat-and-ugly body?" By choosing to define "thin" as beautiful and "round" as ugly, you condemn yourself unnecessarily to a painful fate. Choosing to define "round" as beautiful is just as easy. Women are round! The average dress size in America is 14 to 16. Few women look like the anorectic fashion models on which your "thin" aspirations are based.

Think about it. Today, this is the only body you have! How many todays will you trash waiting for that fantasy body of tomorrow?

To be absolutely clear, let's say that for the next 365 days your current weight remains unchanged. On the 366th day, you're magically transformed and placed inside your dream body. Fine. But are you honestly willing to scrap those other precious days, weeks, and months? Are you genuinely willing to deprive yourself of full happiness for yet another year waiting for the Day of Transformation?

It's an awful price to pay. But it's the price you agree to every day that you refuse to accept your body.

Objection 2: "How can I say I'm beautiful when society tells me I'm not?"

Answer: Let me reassure you—I am not naive. I know that our society degrades larger people. As I mentioned earlier, I know that studies show you'll most likely lose out to the thinner but no-better-qualified person on jobs, in school interviews, and in jury trials.

But you have a choice. You can continue to submit to someone else's ideal by once again tormenting and torturing your body; you can continue to have those days when you wake up depressed, frightened, at your wit's end; and you can continue to grouse, grumble, and weep over the incredible injustice. Or, you can determine that all things are *not* equal, summon up some justifiable anger, and declare that you *won't* lose out to the thinner person because you *will* go that extra step to be better. Is it fair? No. But what has grieving and anguishing over this situation gotten you?

Women in our culture have fought for—and made—some exciting inroads (even as you read, more feminist issues are being hotly debated). But there is one area that continues silently and insidiously to taint those hard-won rights and drain those successes of their joy. It's a hidden tyranny that continues to keep women on the edge, "in their place," and inferior: body size. Doesn't it stand to reason that as long as women play along, perpetuate the societal attitude, and actively dislike their physical shapes, fulfillment and well-being will be stifled?

See, there's a basic lie that must be addressed. There is no real entity called society—there's only *you*. *You* are society. Because you buy into the prejudice against larger-than-thin female bodies, the bigotry persists.

Would you allow someone to denigrate your religious beliefs, your

political choices, or your moral views? Hardly. But if that same someone comments, "You could stand to lose a few pounds," you'll quickly
nod your head in shamed agreement and willingly sacrifice your personal power and your dignity.

Society does not have the power to diminish you unless you choose
to accept the notion that you, at your size, deserve to be put down. If
you're not part of the solution (a person who lovingly accepts her body),
then you are part of the problem.

Objection 3: "Okay, it's fine to tell myself I'm great the way I
am—but what about what everyone else thinks?"

Answer: Teaching the seminars has made me realize that as an
Overeater, you actually believe you're psychic and can read minds.
You're convinced that the thoughts of everyone else are focused just as
yours are, on your stomach, hips, and thighs—that because that's all
you see, that's all *they* see. But here's the catch: Most people are too
busy worrying about themselves and their own lives to give a hoot about
your body. If you happen to be round and someone does deign to notice
your body long enough to shoot it down, believe me, you haven't been
singled out for special criticism. Anyone at any size is fair game for the
fleeting insensitivity of others. (Nancy Reagan has suggested that during her terms as First Lady, some Washington women were hostile to
her because she is a size 4!)

Let me give you another example. A few months ago, my wife and
I joined some friends for dinner—four couples we knew, and one couple we'd recently met. The new woman was a professional model who
frequently appears on magazine covers—5 feet, 8 inches tall, 105
pounds, blonde hair, blue eyes.

As it happened, when the evening drew to an end, the model and
her husband were the first to leave. Immediately, the remaining women
started in: "Can you believe *she's* a model?" one stated. "Her face is
nowhere!" said another. "She must be a model," a third chimed in, "she's
so ordinary looking that makeup artists can use her face like a blank
canvas!" The beat went on.

Do you get the idea? If people are so inclined, they can always
come up with a few nasty remarks to bandy about, no matter how
you look.

In a subsequent seminar, my wife heard me repeating this incident
and informed me that while my observation was valid, I had missed
the major point for indicting the model. See objection 4.

Objection 4: "I'd feel like a fool if I acted as if I were beautiful
when I know people are thinking how fat I am."

Answer: Let's return to that infamous dinner. In truth, that night, the model was acting the picture of haughtiness, superiority, and affectation. The negative opinions and reactions expressed by the other women had nothing to do with her looks. They were occasioned by her attitude. This is important: As a victim of the Diet Mentality, you don't realize the power you have over others' opinions! Although by societal standards, that model was absolutely gorgeous, like Gloria, she might have felt wretched (for personal reasons), insecure (meeting new people), and perhaps even "fat" (she's a woman!). If you choose to feel fat and ugly, your behavior will reflect it and others will treat you accordingly. If you choose to feel good about yourself, that attitude will shine through and others will find you attractive.

Jennie and Eve are prime examples of these two starkly contrasting attitudes. Jennie is a woman in her early sixties, of medium height, 155 to 160 pounds. She came to a seminar convinced that her weight was responsible for her terrible life—particularly her relationships with men—which was a series of disasters. Jennie told the group story after story of emotionally abusive lovers who had used her weight to torment her, then left, citing her "fatness" as their excuse.

Until she came to the seminar, she had never heard women at her size (and much larger) tell of enjoying warm, nurturing relationships with men. She was amazed that none of these women had experienced similarly cruel treatment or heard similarly brutal weight remarks. The information came as an epiphany.

Feeling as bad as she did about her weight, Jennie frequently attached herself to abusive men—she believed she had no choice, they were all she deserved, they were all she could get. To ensure that these men would know that she *knew* she was fat, she focused her attention on her weight. Armed with the information she willingly provided, they, too, focused on her weight and used that Achilles heel to attack her. It wasn't until the seminar that Jennie realized she had given them the ammunition, then sucked in the comments and the abuse and made it all "real."

Eve, on the other hand, is a totally different story. She came across to the group as a "well put together," attractive, bright, powerful woman. Despite the fact that she weighed about 100 pounds more than Jennie, she wasn't viewed as a fat person.

Radiating ingeniousness and intelligence, Eve, who is from Washington, D.C., where there are seven women for every man, made a comment about herself that rattled the group consciousness. She said that when she was single, if she happened to walk into a party and saw one attractive man surrounded by six other Washington women, she had no doubt: She'd be the one he'd make the move on.

There wasn't a soul in the room who didn't believe her.

Objection 5: "If I accept my body, I'll lose my motivation to change it."

Answer: Remember—thinness doesn't motivate! On the other hand, self-acceptance gives you the freedom to act, and that *will* motivate you to nurture yourself. (Think back to the analogy of the unwanted candlestick versus the beloved vase—which will receive your tender care?)

Acceptance is a breeder of motivation. For instance, this year, in order to spend twice as much time in the gym as I did last year, I get up an hour earlier than I used to. No, I'm not motivated to get to the gym because I believe my body is defective. I'm motivated by the pleasure I received from looking and feeling so good last year. This year, I wanted to double that experience. The more you *like* your appearance, the better you care for yourself. The more you care for yourself, the better you like your appearance. It's a proven cycle of success.

Objection 6: "If I love my body, won't I have to give up my hopes and dreams of being thin?"

Answer: There's an irony that victims of the Diet Mentality inevitably miss: The world is so busy with its own concerns, and so oblivious to your weight, it actually will allow you to pursue and achieve all of your goals—without losing an ounce!

If you pursue your goals with an attitude of entitlement, the world will not dare to sneer at you because you're round. The only one who spouts that damning view is you! (In chapter 7, you're going to learn exactly how to reach your goals—right now!)

Objection 7: "In the past, when I accepted my body the way it was, my weight went up!"

Answer: You never really accepted your body. You merely resigned yourself to it and acted from a sense of defeat. Defeat is a painful feeling. It perpetuates self-loathing; it breeds neglect. And it doesn't stop there. When you feel disgusting to yourself, you're driven to find something to soothe, and, of course, food is the quickest remedy. Immediate food will subdue your feelings of disgust; more food will narcotize them. To get that food drug working immediately, you'll eat in the absence of your Hunger Signals and beyond your Satisfaction Signals. You'll put on excess weight, and then hate yourself again—this time with new intensity.

Objection 8: "I can't wear decent clothes at this size. Pretty clothes stop at size 13."

Answer: Quite simply, this is wrong! You've avoided shopping for too long. Some time ago, designers realized that the average woman's size is 14 to 16, and for several years they have been producing smart, fashionable clothes in larger sizes.

This particular objection is fostered by a reluctance to adorn your body at its current size. "Why waste the money on clothes for this body when I intend to replace it with a smaller one?" goes the thinking. When you hate your body, you avoid looking at the beautiful clothes (why make yourself feel worse?), and you avoid shopping for clothes in your size (if they fit, they must be ugly). You'll buy shoes, scarves, and bags, but if it's made to slip over your stomach, hips, or arms, you'll slink off in a state of massive denial.

Check out your local department store and the new boutiques specially designed for high-fashion larger sizes.

Objection 9: "If you have a problem like high blood pressure, you have to lose weight."

Answer: This objection is tricky. There are two types of Overeaters who bring it up. The first type has grown comfortable using the physical condition or "disability" as an excuse to continue suffering about weight. Interestingly, when the physical condition is resolved but no substantial weight loss has occurred, their emotional pain does not abate. In effect, the "condition" justifies their need to obsess about weight.

The second type of Overeater is genuinely concerned about health/ weight issues. (As you'll read later, with the exception of the highest percentiles, I totally disagree with the notion that a higher weight is a risk factor. See chapter 10.)

In reviewing the studies, it appears that *overeating and weight fluctuations* are the culprits promoting the health risks associated with overweight. I can tell you story after story of seminar graduates who began to respond to their Body Signals, then visited their physicians, and without having yet lost their first ounce, found that their cholesterol levels or blood sugar levels or blood pressures had moved from high to normal.

If you have a "weight-related" problem, you probably don't need to lose weight. You do need to listen to your Body Signals and eat nutritiously.

Objection 10: "Intellectually, I agree—I should accept my body as it is. But I don't really *feel* beautiful."

Answer: All I ask is that you choose to *accept* your body as fine and beautiful, to appreciate its appearance, to feel love for it—*for 2 minutes!*

That's right. For 2 minutes!

Let me explain. Up to now, you believed you had no choice in how you felt about your body. Since your body does not conform to your arbitrarily set standards, *you must dislike it.*

Absence of choice means absence of personal power means absence of freedom. You must understand that you have a choice!

Today, for the entire day, the body you have is the only body you can have. (If a bomb drops right now, believe it—you're going out in this one!)

Since you now know that you created the feeling of dislike, I'm asking you to channel the same energy into creating a new standard for yourself. For today, you're going to choose your appearance the way it is as your standard of beauty. Just for today! Correction: Not even for the day—for 2 minutes!

Why 2 minutes? To demonstrate to yourself that you can create your own experience. By dealing with the "now," you don't have to concern yourself with worries about your future body. Just enjoy this body for 2 minutes to prove to yourself that you can make this vital, self-beneficial choice and actually change your feelings.

You know the cliché about riding a bicycle: Once you've done it, shaky though it may feel, you know you are capable of doing it again. Acceptance works the same way.

I'm not so obtuse that I think you will never want a thinner body. But there's a crucial distinction to be made: You must get to the point where you don't *need* a smaller body.

If you can create that experience for 2 minutes now, then you can recreate that feeling any time you choose.

Making This Permanent

At a certain point in the seminars, after all the participants have actually created a true feeling of love and acceptance for their bodies, I ask for a volunteer spokesperson to engage in a conversation.

Steve: How does the acceptance feel?

Participant: It feels better than hating my appearance!

Steve: Then why don't you look happy?

Participant: I'm not sure . . . .

Further discussion illuminates the remaining doubts: "How real is this feeling?" "Why does it seem to come and go from minute to minute?" "How can I recreate this under the stress of living in the real world?" "Will I get used to this strange sensation of actually feeling good about my body?"

The questions are valid.

Creating a permanent acceptance that engenders freedom and great feeling is similar to creating firm abdominal muscles that bespeak discipline and strength. They don't simply appear. You must do the sit-ups or leg raises—you must take action and exercise the muscles.

Creating permanent acceptance and providing yourself with the motivation to listen to your Body Signals consistently is the same. You must exercise the muscle! You must demonstrate your acceptance every day. In other words, you must "fake it until you make it."

"Fake it until you make it" doesn't mean pretend. "I fake it every time I put on a bathing suit," one woman exclaimed. "On the outside I look like I'm having a wonderful time. But inside, I'm miserable— I'm still self-conscious about my body."

That's not what I'm talking about.

"Fake it until you make it" means putting yourself back into the center of that 2-minute experience whenever you need it. Recreate the 2 minutes of acceptance and experience it as though it's your authentic feeling.

Think of your 2-minute acceptance experience as a magic cloak. When you need to feel strong, beautiful, and free, you simply fling the "fake-acceptance-until-I-make-acceptance" cloak around your shoulders and recreate the experience.

But remember: Recreating your 2 minutes of acceptance is totally different from pretending you feel acceptance. You can't pretend something you've never actually felt before (at least not in a body you hate).

The "Miracle" Letters

Some people want to respond to their Body Signals to alter their relationship with food. Their interest stops there. Others, however, want to tune in to their Body Signals not only to alter their relationship with food but also to alter their relationships with spouses, careers, finances, sex, and friends. For too long, the failure to love and accept who they are and how they look has dominated and stifled their lives. And, as their attitudes change, their lives begin to blossom.

Seminar graduates often write me letters dramatically detailing the difference acceptance has made in their lives. I call these messages the miracle letters.

One day I received a miracle phone call that clearly demonstrated how "fake it until you make it" can actually change a life.

It was from my mother.

"Fake It" to Success

After decades of dieting, she came to New York from her home near Washington, D.C., and attended the seminar. Months later, she called and told me, "This program has had such an incredible effect on me, I want to make it available to the people of Washington. I'm going to produce the seminars here for you to teach."

Still, although she was definitive and resolute, her Internal Saboteur was acting up: "People will look at you as an overweight, middle-aged woman. People will be turned off," it told her. She decided to ignore the voice and the disastrous images, and do it anyway.

But how to start? She came up with a great idea. Why not approach a newspaper for a free quarter-page ad? (She was so enthused, I didn't want to burst her bubble by pointing out that newspapers operate on revenues!)

The next morning, determined to look terrific (as I think she always does), she dressed, made herself up with extra care, and started driving to the newspaper offices. On the way, her Internal Saboteur started up again: "Are you nuts? Newspapers don't give free ads! Your idea is crazy! Turn around now!"

And again, in spite of the disturbing messages, she continued. Upon arriving at the newspaper offices, she stepped out of the car, threw her shoulders back, stood up straight, and said to herself: "I am a beautiful, powerful woman—and beautiful, powerful women get what they want!"

Fueled by her own determination, she marched into the building and entered the elevator. Upon reaching her floor, she stepped out and passed a well-dressed woman in her midthirties who was walking in carrying a briefcase—and something happened that my mother had never before experienced with a stranger. "Excuse me," the younger woman said, holding the elevator door for a moment. My mother turned around and heard her say, "I just want to tell you that you are one of the most strikingly beautiful women I've ever seen!"

Astonished, delighted, and totally validated, my mother walked into the offices and approached the advertising people with her scheme. When the meeting was over, she ran to the nearest telephone, called me in New York, and said, "This stuff works!"

Did they give her the free quarter-page ad? No. In all honesty, I must tell you she didn't get it. Instead, they gave her a free full-page ad!

When you accept your body exactly as it is today, you'll lose the timidity, the self-consciousness, the less-than-the-rest feeling that drives you to avoid challenge and confrontation. The miracle letters and phone calls prove it over and over.

"Now that I'm feeling feisty again," one seminar graduate wrote, "my life is going so great, I actually *want* people to mess with me."

You can believe her. Acceptance works!

Chapter 7

Getting What You Want with the Body You're In

Why wait until you're thinner
to live the life you want?
Can you come up with one good reason?

Two close friends, Kathy and Jane (both victims of the Diet Mentality), are sitting in a restaurant engaged in a conversation about their lives.

"I wish my body were more toned," Kathy is saying. "It would be wonderful to walk into a store and actually pick out the clothes I want." Jane nods sympathetically. "If I got my body into shape, maybe then I could also get Bob to bring a little romance back into our marriage," she states. "I've forgotten the meaning of great sex . . . you know what I mean?" Jane nods again, and says, "Oh, yeah."

"And I wish I had more confidence in expressing my feelings," Kathy continues. "Life would certainly improve at the office . . . I'm just not comfortable with those group presentations. Actually, Jane, I also think I'd spend a lot more positive time with my children." Kathy pauses here and sighs.

"Well, I guess if I want to feel confident and comfortable, I'd need to be able to look in a mirror and like what I see. You know, if I didn't have all this fat, I'd have the self-esteem I need to get some control in my life. I'd sure feel more content. I'd be free of my obsession with weight; I'd be in control of food. I'd be happy." Jane nods again, very knowingly.

Throughout this discussion, Jane nods her head in a continuous motion of understanding. Curiously, when Kathy and Jane finish their

103

talk and go their separate ways, both believe that intimate information has been exchanged.

In point of fact, it hasn't. Jane has not a shred of an idea of what Kathy actually wants! Kathy merely tossed Jane a bunch of conceptual thoughts—general, unfocused, and nonspecific. And Kathy doesn't know that if she wants to produce results, *these thoughts are useless!*

The diet industry loves to eavesdrop on just such intimate discussions. It's easy to exploit the unfocused thinking of people trapped in the Diet Mentality. Like Kathy, Chronic Dieters believe that thinness will provide for all their wants. Chances are, you also want the same things Kathy said she wants. But do you honestly believe you know what she wants? Chances are that like Jane, you have no idea what Kathy actually wants—and you are just as unclear about what you want.

A Proving Quiz

Let me prove my point. Chronic Dieters often speak in vague concepts that may contain poetic allure but no functional rewards. If you believe you're different from them, take a shot at this quiz. (Before you begin, however, there is one rule. Your answers may *not* include these three words: *feel, know,* or *see*—unfocused words that provide no functional information.) Go ahead.

1. How would you know that your body is toned?
2. How do you know which clothes make you feel beautiful?
3. What is something you would be doing if you had romance?
4. What is something you would be doing if you had great sex?
5. What is something you would do if you had confidence?
6. If you were to express your feelings, what would you say?
7. How would you know that it's time to like what you see when you look in a mirror? (The numbers on the scale and your dress size don't count.)
8. What is something you would be doing that would let you know it was time to be happy?
9. If you freed yourself of your obsession with food, what would you replace your obsession with?
10. If you were in control of food, what food would you eat? (The words *healthy* and *nutritious* don't count.)

Tough quiz, isn't it? Were you able to answer these questions without using the forbidden words? Until you can, you have almost no chance of getting what you want.

"I Don't Want Cereal"

Nor do you have any chance of getting what you want through negative statements. Let's suppose you walk into your kitchen one morning and your mate says, "I'm going to make breakfast for you, honey. What do you want?"

"I don't want cereal," you reply.

Pretty silly answer, right? If your spouse looks perplexed, it's no wonder. Yet, "I don't want cereal," is the way most victims of the Diet Mentality define their desires. *You attempt to define what you want by describing what you don't want!*

When I ask seminar participants what they want, I usually receive two types of replies. Either nonspecific answers (confidence, self-esteem, happiness—like Kathy's list) or what isn't wanted (like cereal). Their answers to the proving quiz look something like this.

1. I would know that my body is toned if I *didn't* have these rolls of fat.
2. I know clothes make me feel beautiful when they *don't* show my bulges.
3. If I had romance, I *wouldn't* sit alone while my husband watches television when he could be with me.
4. If I had great sex, I *wouldn't* get uptight about having my body looked at.
5. If I had confidence, I *wouldn't* worry about what people thought about my behavior.

Do you get the point?

The Lightning Theory of Attainment

Toni, a woman in her early forties, attended a seminar, and during one of the exercises, told the group, "I want to be happy." For seven years, she had been in an unhappy marriage. A stay-at-home housewife who wanted to be a businesswoman, her social life revolved around her husband's friends, none of whom she enjoyed. Toni felt uninvolved in—and cut off from—the world around her.

A year before attending the seminar, she divorced her husband and started her own business (it was now grossing three times its projected income). She had made many new friends, was dating frequently, and had her pick of men. Not only was she socially active, she had also become involved in meaningful community projects.

After Toni told us this story, I repeated it to her and then asked what she needed to be happy. A look of shock appeared on her face. Her hands flew up to the sides of her head. "Oh, my God," she exclaimed incredulously. "I *am* happy!"

Every seminar participant claims to want confidence, self-esteem, and happiness. But like Toni, even if all the components were present and in place in their lives, they still might not realize they already had gotten what they wanted.

Victims of the Diet Mentality operate by what I call the Lightning Theory of Attainment. The mechanism is simple. Overeating Dieters believe that all they need is to want something like confidence or happiness in their lives and it will magically zap them. Perhaps it will occur on the street. As they amble along deep in a private reverie, a bolt of magic lightning will suddenly strike them, and instantaneously, like a character in "Star Trek," they will be beamed up to a new life. Goodbye former meek, mild-mannered, unhappy self. Hello assertive, self-assured, happy, super self. The lightning will transform their lives.

Again, the diet industry loves this theory. It counts on your belief in the Lightning Theory of Attainment. While you're waiting for the magic bolt to strike, you're ripe for their rip-offs. You're a pushover. You can be easily enticed into believing that any new diet product appearing on the market will indeed zap you with that bolt of lightning, rescue you from despair, and beam you up to happiness.

Act First! Your Feelings Will Follow

To keep the record straight, let me give you a definition of happiness: "Feeling you are in control of your life and taking action consistent with your feeling."

Toni fit this definition. She was in control and taking action in every important area of her life. (That's why I suspected she was happy before she did.)

Do you remember the section called "Learn—Do—Feel" in chapter 5 (see page 82)? I'll help to refresh your memory. Overeaters wait until they *feel* different before they *act*. As a result, they usually spend more time waiting for their feelings to change than they do acting. To produce the results you're after, you must reverse that process: You must act first!

Feelings are a result of actions. At best, waiting for your feelings to change is dicey—they may change, or they may not. At worst, waiting for your feelings to change is about the same as trashing your life. If Toni had waited for her feelings to change before acting on her desires, she might still be sitting at home with her husband, growing more despondent with each passing year. Instead, she began to move, and as she moved, her feelings changed. She began to take charge of her life in the same way a happy person takes charge, and the feelings caught up with her. (Toni didn't realize she was happy because her self-definition got in the way. When she removed it—and it only took a moment!—she realized this is what happiness looks like, this is how happiness feels.)

Changing the Circumstances of Your Life

How do you gain control of your life? Many participants walk into the seminars feeling trapped by their circumstances—professionally stifled by family responsibilities, frustrated by long, hard hours of work supporting families, restrained by physical ailments, disappointed by sexually unresponsive spouses, trapped in dead-end jobs, reined-in socially, and most of all, limited in all areas of their lives by "fat."

By the end of the seminar, these same people know that they do have the capacity to change their lives.

Not by magic. Not by lightning. But by learning some simple techniques that bring about a change in attitude.

It's the Details That Count!

Quickly—which of the following would be more useful to controlling your weight? (1) Planning and implementing a change to nutritious foods or (2) cleaning your messy closets (or basement or garage).

The answer is (2). Cleaning your messy closets is much more closely related to gaining a sense of control than changing to nutritious foods. Here's why.

You know the feeling of control. You've cleaned out the closets, thrown out empty shoe boxes, arranged the winter clothes up front and stored the summer clothes in back. You've accomplished what you set out to do. Cleaning a closet is a detail you can control and a detail that gives you a feeling of control. (You may also remember that cleaning a closet has a ripple effect on other areas in your life.)

Many Overeaters, particularly women, tend to be broad, visionary thinkers. Like Kathy, they can visualize lofty ideals and happy endings; they can see the hero and heroine stroll off into the sunset. But when it comes to filling in the details, the vision goes blank.

To gain control of food (and other areas of your life), you must look at the details and begin to tend to them. Although you already know a lot about the business of details, you just haven't applied that same thinking to your relationship to food, weight, and your Body Signals. (By the way, changing to nutritious foods is not a detail—it's a project. Manage the details and the projects will follow.)

Your Life—The Book

Putting the concept of managing into action isn't as easy as it may seem. The Diet Mentality thrives on shortcuts. That's why I ask Overeaters to project themselves three years into the future and visualize their hopes and dreams already fulfilled. Then I suggest they pretend they're writing their autobiographies and ask them to speak about their new lives.

Interestingly, while enthusiasm runs high, no one fulfills the assignment on the first try. Everyone writes the chapter titles, but no one supplies the details. As a result, their autobiographies look like a conglomeration of headings.

Chapter 1: I Gained Control of Food
Chapter 2: I Eat Nutritiously
Chapter 3: I Have Self-Confidence
Chapter 4: My Relationship with My Mate Is Wonderful
Chapter 5: My Children Are Growing Up Healthy and Happy

Your Life—The Movie

Their next task is to pretend they're the writer and the director of a movie that will capture the essence of their particular lifestyle and to select the actor or actress who will play their lives—many pick Meryl Streep. Try it for a moment.

It's the first scene, you're directing Meryl, and you ask her to demonstrate your new self-confidence. No, you can't just say, "Meryl, act confident!" It's too vague. What is she doing? What is she saying? Who is in the scene with her? For the scene to work, you must provide the details.

From Out of Control to In Control

Vagueness will not produce results. Generalities are useless. If it takes either adjectives or adverbs to state what it is that you want, like the chapter headings in *Your Life—The Book,* your desires will be too hazy.

And again, it's equally nonproductive to define what you want by what you don't want: "I'd like to be free of _____. I'd like to lose _____. I'd like to rid myself of _____. I'd like to stop _____." Those are the words of dieters! By employing these useless phrases, you'll continue to program yourself to remain out of control and to hang on to everything you wish to be free of. What you resist, persists. With some simple changes, however, most of your wants will become real and within your control.

The Arithmetic of Success

Right now, your goal is to feel in control around food. That feeling is produced through actions. So if the chapter heading in your autobiography is "I Gained Control of Food," you'll need to add up some details (actions) to produce the feeling. Your details could look something like this:

"In the last six months, I did the following:

- Prepared a list before I went grocery shopping—and stuck to it
- Ate before I went grocery shopping
- Introduced brown rice into my diet and ate at least four servings a week
- Read a nutrition book
- Went to a restaurant x number of times and had only conversation after the main course (or left after the main course) 80 percent of the time

- Ate fruit for dessert 75 percent of the time
- Ate a maximum of 20 ounces of red meat a week
- Ate fried food a total of three times
- Averaged 15 servings of vegetables a week
- Felt stressed, depressed, or bored 50 times and responded with a phone call to a friend, a soothing shower massage, or a walk 45 times
- Attended two weddings at which I ate cake and hors d'oeuvres and drank champagne, and later, after both events, told myself it was fine
- Ate junk food a total of six times"

Looking at this list of accomplished details, you may conclude that it's now time for you to feel in control of food. Then again, you may decide that accomplishing half of the items on the list would give you that feeling. Or maybe you'd need to add several more items to produce the results. The point is that you must determine what specific actions *you* must take to build the feelings you want to have.

Stating What You Want

When you examine the language of successful people who repeatedly get what they want, something extremely interesting comes to light. They state what they want in a special way. Vague concepts like happiness and confidence don't muddle their sentences. Instead, their words, like their intentions, are clear. How do they pull this off? By sticking to these seven simple steps:

Step 1: Be Specific

General I Want:	Specific I Want:
A toned body	A flat stomach; space between my thighs when I walk; the ability to bend over and touch my toes with my knees straight
Beautiful clothes	Pastel colors; a wide belt; midthigh-length skirt; a blouse that shows cleavage
To express my feelings	To tell my mother my weight is none of her business

General I Want:	Specific I Want:
Self-esteem	To walk into my class reunion with my shoulders back and a smile on my face, as I start up conversations with my former classmates

Step 2: Be Positive

Negative I Want:	Positive I Want:
To stop thinking of food	To think of food only when I'm hungry
To get rid of my obsession with weight	To throw my scale away
To stop losing my temper	To take a deep breath before I react

Step 3: Use Action Words (Verbs)— Not Emotion Words

Emotion I Want:	Action I Want:
To feel in control of food	To eat four, five, or six bites of dessert and stop when I'm satisfied
To feel good about myself	To meet with friends at least once a week for lunch, dinner, a party, or an outing
To like what I see in the mirror	To look in the mirror from the neck down and state out loud, "You look great!"
To enjoy sex	To initiate sexual activities at least half the time

Step 4: Put Your Desires in a Precise Context: What? Who? When? Where? Avoid Adjectives and Adverbs

Vague I Want:	Precise I Want:
More confidence	To offer my opinions to my boss when she's deciding a work-policy issue, and have her listen
More control in social situations	To walk up to people I want to talk to at parties, look them in the eye, stand up straight, start a conversation, and tell myself that they want to talk to me
To spend more positive time with my children	To spend at least ½ hour a day with each child, reading, talking, or playing a game
To procrastinate less	To clean my house once every two weeks; to finish my tax returns by April 5th; to fix the dripping kitchen faucet by next Sunday

Step 5: Know What's in Your Control

Someone Else Controls I Want:	I Control I Want:
My husband to bring me flowers	To ask my husband to bring me flowers
My son to receive all A's and B's	To spend ½ hour every night reviewing my son's homework with him
My daughter to stop using drugs	To see a counselor and learn what I can do to help my daughter stop using drugs

Someone Else Controls I Want:	I Control I Want:
My boss to stop yelling at me when he gets upset	To tell my boss that I will not tolerate his raising his voice to me

Step 6: Quantify: How Much? How Long? How Many? By When?

Not Quantifiable I Want:	Quantifiable I Want:
To be an Instinctive Eater	To eat when my body is hungry at least 90 percent of the time
To exercise regularly	To exercise at least ½ hour three times a week
To be financially independent	To increase my annual income by 20 percent
To feel confident at parties	To choose at least four people with whom to start a conversation at every party I attend
To have a firm body	To pick ten weight lifting or Nautilus exercises and increase the weight on each of them by at least 10 pounds within a year
To have a better position	To become manager of my division next year

Are you keeping track? So far, your desires must be specific, positive, employ action words, be placed in a specific context, remain within your control, and be quantifiable.

Step 7: Do a Balance Check

This is the all-important step for determining whether you're willing to give something up to get what you want. Right now, although you may feel awful, terrific, or both, we could call your life balanced. (I make this assumption because you are surviving, probably by employing some interesting survival techniques—bingeing may be one of them. You may not like it, but it has served your purposes. Bad as the bingeing feels, you *are* still alive.)

If we're going to define your life as balanced, that means you have to be careful about making changes. You want to make sure that pursuing what you want and getting it won't throw the balance off.

To square your want with your willingness to have, you must learn to do a balance check. That means you must assess honestly, if not ruthlessly, what your current behavior provides for you and what your desire might provide. What do you win by perpetuating the old behavior? What will you lose by achieving the new goal?

When your assessment is completed, compare your present life (without the goal) to what your future life will be (with the goal achieved), and decide which you prefer.

I'll give you a personal example. In 1986, I decided I wanted to run a marathon. To undergo the proper training, there were certain activities I'd have to give up—sleeping late on weekends, eating dinner at the customary time, maintaining my usual patient schedule, keeping evenings free to relax at home with a book.

I decided the marathon wasn't worth it. I wasn't willing to give up those activities. Since I wasn't committed to completing the project, I didn't begin it.

In 1987, I decided to run the marathon and, again, balanced my dream of accomplishing it with the sacrifices of training. This time I was clear that the sacrifices were worth it and I was willing to make them. I spent the year undergoing the training I needed to fulfill my goal.

A Perfect Example: To Binge or Not to Binge

Let's consider bingeing. You're interested in controlling your weight permanently and you begin by setting a goal: "For at least the next three years, I will eat at least 90 percent of the time when I feel a Hunger Signal in my body."

Sounds great. Look at all the benefits you'll gain: You'll be in control of food; you'll lose any excess pounds; you'll experience a new sense of health; you'll feel better about yourself; you'll wear new, fashionable clothes. What could be wrong with that?

Plenty.

Until you've figured out what you're giving up to achieve your goals, it's better not to set any goals.

Bingeing and fat provide for many of your needs. While giving them up may offer you that wonderful list of benefits, they may not be as valuable as what you'll lose.

For example, bingeing and fat provide:

• A blanket solution for managing stress
• An immediate outlet for soothing painful emotions
• A narcotic for lulling emotional pain
• A method for avoiding sexual tensions
• An excuse for failure
• A source of instant pleasure

Are you willing to give this up? Make your assessment. Which set of benefits will you choose—those that have already proven effective, or those that you may or may not achieve by making the promise?

Realizing Your Desires

By using the seven steps starting on page 110 to state what they want, successful people accomplish two things: They make their desires clear and doable, and they determine the difference between what they merely want (*e.g.,* the 1986 marathon) and what they're actually willing to have or pursue (*e.g.,* the 1987 marathon).

As soon as successful people decide they're willing to "go for it," their next step is to convert their "want" into a promise or commitment. They then set the wheels in motion to make that commitment become a reality.

I'll show you how.

Programming Yourself to Succeed: The Time Machine

So far, you've clearly stated your goal, and you know that you're willing to have what you want. Now you're going to make a commitment: "For at least three years, I will eat at least 90 percent of the time in response to my Body Signals."

It's still not all clear sailing. You haven't dealt with the obstacles yet, and you're going to be confronted with what seems like an endless series of them. (This is true of just about any important goal.)

How do you ensure that you'll overcome these obstacles and stick to your commitment?

First, it's important that you develop a safety net by making your new commitment known to a friend, family member, or group who will hold you accountable and be there to support you should you go into "breakdown."

Next, you climb into what I call the mental time machine and travel three years into the future. Project yourself forward and stop there for a few minutes. Take some time with this exercise. Look around—see what you've accomplished by eating in response to your Body Signals, see just how you accomplished it. Then return to the present.

The mental time machine changes your mindset. Instead of making plans and hoping they'll bear fruit, you mentally live out the deed before beginning it. Projecting into the future gives you a head start. You're privy to what the journey will look like, as well as a sense of what obstacles will pop up and how you'll handle them. When you actually do launch your plans and obstacles arise that didn't emerge on your mental time trip, you won't feel as flustered: You'll feel confident you can handle them because you've already proved your capability and readiness on the mental journey.

This is how you program yourself to succeed. The mental time machine will program you from committing to planning, from planning to doing, from doing to adjusting, and from adjusting to having.

Three years from now, in retelling how you achieved your goal, your story might sound something like this.

Back to the Future

"I picked up a book called *The Body-Signal Secret* and after reading it, promised myself I'd eat at least 90 percent of my meals in response to my body's Hunger Signals and Satisfaction Signals. The next morning, I began waiting for my body to give me a Hunger Signal. I waited all day. Nothing happened. 'I can't hack this!' I declared, and ate a meal anyway.

"Afterward, I started berating myself: 'There's another one of your good intentions that lasted all of a day—you've failed again.' I caught myself in the act. 'Wait a minute,' I said. 'Didn't you read, "Turn failure into feedback and learn lessons from the obstacles rather than letting them defeat you?" Yes. Okay. Let me get off my back and give it another try tomorrow.' That decision made me feel a renewed sense of purpose. Instead of failing, I had overcome my first obstacle—the desire to give up.

"Over the next few days, every so often, I began to notice a sensation in my stomach, but it was confusing. It seemed that sometimes food made the sensation disappear, but at other times, I just wasn't clear what was happening.

"During those first two or three weeks, I frequently found myself eating because it was mealtime. 'You're blowing your promise!' I'd tell myself. Then I'd answer, 'No, get off it! This is *not* some diet you've blown. Give yourself a break—you've been dieting and bingeing for years; you're only a beginner at this Body Signal thing. You just have to keep trying.'

"The internal conversation helped: I realized I had overcome another major obstacle to success—the desire to beat myself up.

"I don't remember the exact day, but one morning I woke up with an empty feeling in my stomach. 'No doubt about it,' I smiled to myself, 'I'm definitely experiencing a Hunger Signal!'

"Up to this point, I was also having trouble with my Satisfaction Signal. This thing called satisfaction seemed like such a mystery: I still wanted to continue eating everything set before me. To outsmart myself, I deliberately made it a point to always leave something on my plate. (Another obstacle managed.)

"As I began to tune in to my Hunger Signals, I realized why satisfaction was so difficult. Satisfaction is the absence of hunger, but since I frequently put food in my mouth when I wasn't hungry, I had no way of knowing when I was satisfied. I couldn't get the idea of absence of hunger. However, as my Hunger Signal became clearer, my Satisfaction Signal seemed to catch up.

"As a matter of fact, my new-found clarity caused a new set of problems. I found myself getting hungry at work when food was unavailable. A contingency plan was instantly launched. I began to keep rice cakes and almond butter in my desk drawer, and brought two pieces of fruit to work each day. While cooking dinner for my family, I also found myself hungry and frequently caught myself nibbling. To plan for these moments, I started eating a small snack in the late afternoon. It took the edge off of my hunger without spoiling my appetite for dinner.

"After several weeks, I experienced a joyous moment that almost turned into disaster. Sitting on the edge of the bed, I pulled on a pair of panty hose, but when I stood up, they sagged to my ankles! I must have lost a lot of weight, I exulted, and slipping back into the Diet

Mentality, I climbed onto the scale. I'd only lost a few pounds. Suddenly, it didn't matter that my mirrors, my clothes, and my friends told me I was looking slim and trim, or that my exercising had converted fat into muscle and that muscle is heavier than fat. What did matter was that after all those weeks, the scale only registered the loss of a lousy few pounds! I was miserable.

"'Enough of this Body Signal business!' I declared. 'I'm going back to a regular old diet and lose some serious weight.' Determined, I spent the next several days preparing for my forthcoming deprivation the way I always had in the past—bingeing my brains out on junk food. (Clearly, I was experiencing a state of 'breakdown.')

"What happened next? I remembered reading that a promise can be extremely difficult to keep unless you make it known to someone who will hold you accountable and be there to support you. 'Okay,' I muttered miserably and thought of my sister, my chosen safety net. When I called her and explained what was happening to me, she was terrific! She reminded me that the scale was my enemy, that diets have always made me fatter, that I looked great, that I had said I felt healthy, and that for the first time in my life, I was at peace around food. That call turned me around.

"I realized I had followed the three-step formula for getting out of 'breakdown,' and it had actually worked. First, I had acknowledged I was breaking my commitment. Second, I had gotten the support I needed from my sister. And finally, I had now recommitted to my promise.

"Instead of wallowing in the defeat of a blown commitment, I felt the pride and renewed strength of another obstacle overcome.

"Over the following three years, I encountered many more obstacles, but they became progressively easier to overcome. For instance, it became easier to ask for the check instead of the dessert menu, to put the family's leftovers in the garbage instead of in my mouth, to limit my emotional binge eating to individual incidents rather than days and weeks, to sit with people who were eating when I wasn't hungry and feel no obligation to join them, to develop a take-it-or-leave-it attitude toward sweets.

"In time, my focus on food became minimal. I had developed a new perspective and had left my old habits behind me. I remembered reading about an ex-bulimic named Beth who had dramatically changed her life, and used her experience to boost me along.

"Eventually, I found that I was no longer focused on what I *didn't* want to do. I was focused on the present and the future—what I *did* want to do—and my life, like Beth's, was dramatically changed."

Beth's Story: Moving Forward Forever

Beth had been a bulimic for 25 years. I saw her 18 months after she had attended a seminar. She told me that her last bulimic episode had taken place one year previously. (At this writing, she's gone 5 years without an episode.) Married to a loving husband, Beth has a bright teenage daughter, and since attending the seminar, a successful consulting business from which she commands high fees and a roster of many celebrated clients.

How did she kick bulimia? Not by forcing herself to stop the bingeing and purging. She kicked it by filling her life with so many engaging pursuits and activities, there was no room to deal with such a time-consuming eating disorder. Her focus is forward, on living her life—not backward, on the specter of bulimia.

Backward focus is anathema for people who want to rid themselves of a habit. With your attention focused on the unwanted habit, failure is inevitable. "Today I won't binge." "Today I won't smoke." "Today I won't gamble." "Today I won't drink." These are all backward-focused statements. When you actively resist your impulse to binge, smoke, gamble, or drink, your emphasis is on the past, that which is behind you—the negative habit. It's easy to see that backward focus basically programs you to fail.

"I will stop bingeing" is a backward-focused negative statement that has no power to produce results. No single declaration can function as a catch-all for a multitude of events.

Let me explain.

Binges are not single events. Each binge is an event in its own right. If you're going to stop bingeing, a blanket alternative won't work, but an individual alternative response for each binge will.

For example, let's say you binge three times a week. One alternative to bingeing won't help. Each year you'd binge 156 times, so you would need 156 alternatives! If you're operating on backward focus, that's a lot of binges to resist!

Forward focus shifts the perspective. A constant focus on what nurtures and supports you will basically program you to succeed. When those 156 moments emerge, you'll be too busy living your life to be excited by bingeing.

To control a habit, don't resist it—simply ignore it. When the impulse hits, don't use your good energy to oppose it, use it to jump into the next engaging, nurturing activity on your slate. The more you fill your life with that which nurtures, engages, and pleases, the less room you have for the struggle against succumbing.

Getting What You Want: A Summary

1. State what you want specifically, positively, using action verbs. Place your desire in a precise context—What? Who? When? Where? Avoid adjectives and adverbs. Keep your desire within your control. Quantify it: How much? How long? How many? By when? And before you commit to your goal, do a balance check to make sure the price is worth it.
2. Do the arithmetic. Determine what series of deeds and actions will produce the desired feeling and begin adding them up. Remember: The details (actions) precede feeling.
3. Once you're clear about what you want, find out if you're willing to have it. (The best evidence of your willingness will come from writing it down. There's a saying: "If it's not written, it's not real.")
4. If you've decided that you are willing to have it in your life and you're ready to make a commitment, then project yourself mentally three years into the future. While you're there, look around. See what you accomplished and how you accomplished it. Be sure to include the obstacles you overcame. It will help you to stick to your commitment.
5. Then take action. And expect to fall flat on your face. When that happens, don't label your attempt a failure. Turn failure into feedback and use it. For example, if your goal is to control bingeing, you might wake up one morning and realize you've been bingeing nonstop for the last two weeks. Don't tell yourself you've failed! Tell yourself that you hit an obstacle. Look for the lesson to be learned from that setback, note it well, then recommit to your goal and move on armed with new information.
6. Make sure you make your promise known to a person or group who will hold you accountable and support you when you fall into "breakdown."
7. Finally, the essential, underlying truth: *You must admit that you can do what you want and have what you want with the body you're in— without having to lose a single ounce!*

Chapter 8

Women of Size Speak Out

*The object is not to stop **wanting** to be thin but to stop **needing** to be thin.*

I'd like you to meet Glenda, Leah, Carolyn, Joanne, Sue, and Carol, all Lighten Up graduates who have the Body-Signal concept. As they'll tell you, it has changed their lives.

Glenda: When you start viewing your body as your friend, you stop all the mental torture and you have a lot of time to actually have a life!

Leah: Here's the bottom line: Accept yourself and treat yourself well—whatever you weigh!

Carolyn: I finally stopped waiting until I got thin to do the things I wanted to do.

Joanne: When I let go of the weight issue—when I'm clear about it—I'm attractive and so much of my life works!

Sue: Since I'm no longer so concerned with what people think about my body, they seem to notice it less!

Carol: One of the major benefits of the program is that it helped me develop a greater self-confidence—you just forget about the weight.

And that's just a sample of what these remarkable women have to say; you'll hear more shortly. But first, let me give you a word of warning: These women are going to tell you some unexpected things. When you're caught in the Diet Mentality, there are only two facts you want to hear from large-size people—how much weight they lost and how fast they lost it. That's not what these women are going to talk about.

If you've been abusing your body with yo-yo dieting for many years (as most of these women have done), it can take a while for your body to realize that you are now responding to its signals. Weight loss is not necessarily fast. And even when these women do lose all the weight they're going to lose, because of their genetic/biochemical makeup, they will still be large.

So even though some of these women have lost varying amounts of weight on the Body-Signal Program, this chapter is not designed to be a testimonial to weight loss. Its aim is to show you how good life can be when you take the focus off of your weight.

These women don't deceive themselves. They worked hard to combat the weight obsession; they worked hard to fight off the cultural message telling them that they should remain obsessed until all the weight comes off; and they continue to work hard at achieving the lives they want.

Their observations are important for two reasons: First, they show you what a full life you can have when you stop putting it on hold while you wait to lose all the weight; second, they show you that you can still "have it all"—even if you're larger than size 6.

When you follow the Body-Signal Program, you'll lose all your excess weight. But no one knows exactly how many pounds that will be. I believe that it's important for you to hear from women who no longer waste their energy waiting until they hit that elusive, magical number. In fact, as you listen to these inspiring women, you may find yourself thinking: I wish *I* could feel that way about myself.

Gail, my co-author, spoke with each woman individually. Here's what she found out.

"As Steve explained, much of what these women say flies in the face of what you've been conditioned to think about weight. As you'll see, they're all vital, intelligent, successful women who have grappled with the 'weight problem' most of their lives. They've now put the weight bogeyman behind them and have turned the Diet Mentality chatter off.

"But rather than have you listen to me talk about them—listen to what they have to say about themselves."

The Women Speak Out

Gail: What made you decide to take the seminar?

Sue: I remember hearing a radio ad for Steve's seminar that said something about not being on a diet, becoming nutritionally sound, and getting on with your life. I went to it because I wanted reinforcement for eating nutritionally and I wanted to develop more self-esteem. I wanted to be involved in *anything* that would promote those results.

Joanne: I decided to go because weight has been the major, if not central, issue of my life. When I was 12 years old, I weighed 160 pounds and that's when I went on my first diet—with pills. For the following 32 years, I tried every diet you can name! In fact, unless I was on a diet, I felt miserable. You know what happened: Each time I tried a new diet and went off it, I gained another 10 pounds, and so I just got fatter and fatter. For all those years, I was either gaining weight or on a .diet to lose it, putting it on or losing some and gaining more again. There was *no* stability.

Carolyn: I had been on the yo-yo dieting thing forever—my whole life—and had come to the end of my rope. I just couldn't do any more diets—they weren't working for me. Basically, I had come to the conclusion that I was damaging my body by all the long fasts. My metabolism had slowed down to practically a screeching halt. I was just barely hanging in there and maintaining my weight at a much higher level than I wanted to be.

        At that point, I had a hard time finding any validation for my experience. At one of those weight-reduction meetings, I told a woman with not nearly the weight problem I had that I was following the prescribed eating plan but

I was still gaining weight. This woman looked at me and said, "I don't believe you."

When I went to Steve's seminar, I wasn't even sure I believed myself anymore. We all do some self-deception and I thought maybe I was really lying to myself. But then he said, "I believe you, and I know why this happened to you!" The seminar validated for me that I wasn't really overeating and that I wasn't a horrible, bad person—and that I wasn't lying!

Glenda: I'd gotten to a point at which I could only lose weight by limiting myself to 900 calories a day! At 1,000 calories I could maintain my weight, but with even as little as 1,100, I'd gain. I was getting very scared. One night, I went to an introductory meeting of Lighten Up to learn about the seminar. A woman stood up and spoke, and since that moment, I've never been the same.

She was a switchboard operator—much larger than I was then. She talked about spending her days in front of the switchboard gobbling up junk food. Then she said she'd done the Lighten Up seminar six months ago. She went on and on about how her life had changed—her irritability was gone, she was no longer withdrawn, her energy levels were way up, she was having a much better time with her friends. While she was speaking, what struck me was that she practically dismissed the fact that in the last six months she had effortlessly lost 45 pounds! Compared to every other good thing that had happened to her, she acted as though the weight loss were just a throwaway benefit!

Gail: Did you have any trouble learning your Body Signals?

Carol: Although I was an Overeater, it didn't take me that long to get in touch with my Hunger Signals. I just followed the program as closely as I could. After a period of responding to my signals religiously, my body didn't want more food and I found that more and more was being left on my plate.

Basically, the Satisfaction Signal came at the same time. If you're concentrating on eating all the right nutrients—the vegetables, the fruits, and the protein-rich foods—your body will be satisfied and you just won't want more. I'm now eating salads without dressing, or sometimes with just a little vinegar—by choice!

The Body Signals work. I don't know how much I weigh—because of the program, I don't weigh myself. I really did throw my scale out—I just don't want to be bothered with it. When I go to the doctor, I don't even look at the number. I've probably lost about 60 pounds all told, but I don't worry about that anymore. I know I've lost weight because my clothes don't fit.

Learning the Body Signals is like anything else in life. If you take the time to make it a habit, then it becomes easier and easier to do.

Joanne: I've been a binger and an Overeater, which means I ate beyond satisfaction. I did have trouble with that signal— you have to keep looking for it and then suddenly, you just know! That's how I learned to eat till I was satisfied. Sometimes I'd find myself eating until I was full. There came a point when I didn't want to go beyond feeling comfortable with the amount of food I was putting in my body.

Looking for the Hunger Signal was a little confusing for me at first, mainly because I was an emotional eater. I never recognized thirst, so every time I was thirsty, I ate, and every time I was tired, I ate! (I'm the kind of person whose psyche keeps pushing.) I was just so compulsive, and I had a need to go, go, go. It didn't matter what I was working on—a painting or some other project—or what time it was: I just didn't want to stop. While I'd be pushing myself, I'd also be eating unconsciously. When I learned to recognize fatigue, if I could afford the time, I'd take a nap during the day instead of eating. The results were really great!

Leah: I'm definitely conscious of when I'm satisfied now. I sometimes ignore the signal, but I'm very aware of it. I go two steps forward and one step back with a lot of things— that's what happens with me. But I know that if you're open to what your body is telling you, the awareness is there. There are still times when I *want* to eat something, but that doesn't mean that I'm hungry. Physical hunger feels a certain way, and I recognize it now. I know if I see something and say, "Oh, that looks good!" it has nothing to do with a Hunger Signal. That has to do with emotional appetite. I really do know now when I'm actually hungry. When I really listen to my Body Signals, I eat less and I do lose weight.

Glenda: Learning your Body Signals is actually very liberating and not very difficult. Hunger is the most confusing, especially if you've always eaten when you're frustrated, as I did, or when you've made a habit of feeling proud of being hungry! But once you figure out what real hunger feels like and where it comes from, you can make the distinction. I've always known my point of satisfaction, but as an Overeater, I just wanted to keep getting the good taste of whatever I was eating into my mouth. I could feel my stomach becoming impacted with food, but didn't want to stop. Now my consciousness tells me: "Enough!" You'd be surprised at what you *don't* eat when you listen to your body.

Gail: What about acceptance—has it worked for you?

Joanne: I don't know exactly how I came to accept myself—something clicked in the seminar. I let go of something I was holding on to and suddenly I was just all right the way I was. It just snapped! Part of it was the concept of eating until you're satisfied. If you're eating that way, you don't get scared anymore about gaining weight. For me, the fear of food lifted. I could buy an ice cream cone, take a bite, and throw the rest away. To this day, I rarely ever finish a meal. Part of it was doing the mirror exercises for 2 minutes every day. I'm free of the weight issue and my life is so much better!

Leah: Acceptance was what I needed. Just to love myself as I am. I'm still working at it.

Sue: I don't have trouble with acceptance now. At some point, I decided this was a stupid, wasteful way to live my life! It didn't happen overnight, but at some point, I just began to stop the conversation in my head and fairly soon afterward, I realized I just wasn't interested in it anymore.

Carolyn: Not too long ago, I was reading a book about compulsive Overeaters, how we deny ourselves and then how that denial creates the compulsion to eat. There was an exercise where they asked you to imagine that you were inhaling dust from another planet that made it impossible—no matter what you ate or didn't eat—to change your body. If you were fat, you were going to stay fat; if you were thin, you were going to stay thin. Whatever you ate—your size would not change. Then they asked: What would you do? Would you continue to starve yourself? The women in this experiment all said, "Let me lose some weight first, then I'll play the game."

That's what happens with the acceptance task. You're asked to accept your body, but the first thing that comes to your mind is: Well, let me lose some weight first, then I'll accept it. I certainly can't accept it like this! Oh, anything but this! But then your consciousness just changes. And it works! I just stopped waiting until I got thin to do the things I wanted to do. Something clicked.

Carol: I did the acceptance exercises right away. At first I looked in the mirror quite often and said, "I love my body!" Now I don't do it anymore because it's really not necessary. The acceptance is there.

Glenda: I distinctly remember when Steve brought up acceptance in the seminar. My first thought was that, if I accept my body, I won't lose weight! For about a week afterward, while I was following the eating guidelines and learning to respond to my signals, I wrestled with that idea. But something was brewing inside me and I found I was looking at my body differently. And I was getting irritable about the calorie and weight discussions among my friends. At that point, I knew the acceptance idea had clicked.

Gail: How did you deal with that inner "conversation"—with the Internal Saboteur?

Joanne: Every single day of my life, I had been obsessed about my weight and my body and the way I looked. In other words, there was rarely a moment when I didn't have a different voice from inside saying: You're too fat. The voice was like a separate mind constantly going and going—no matter *what* was happening.

I also remember that when I did the seminar, there was a famous fashion model in the group who looked fabulous to me. Later, I found out that she was in as much agony over her appearance as the women who weighed 250 pounds.

After I did the seminar, I totally accepted the way I was. And really, that voice just unbelievably disappeared!

Leah: I know that changing that internal tape is extremely important. If I start telling myself something very negative about my body and catch myself, I now say, "Thank you for sharing! But I'm okay as I am."

Sue: I remember a woman, a veteran graduate of the seminar, telling a story of cleaning the house wearing one of her size 44 blouses. She said she caught a glimpse of herself in the mirror and even though she was now a size 14, she went right into the same old internal conversation: "Oh, my God, I look disgusting, I'm awful! I *have* to go shopping, but I'll have to wait until I lose 50 pounds to give myself some incentive!"

When she realized what she was doing, she stopped cold and told herself: "I quit this conversation months ago. I don't have time for it! What am I doing?" That's how I feel now—I'm just not interested in this dialogue!

Now about 90 percent of the time (not *all* the time), the new conversation I have about my body is that it's kind of nice to touch and it's soft and really not so bad. I like to say I have a preference—I'd definitely prefer to be a size 10. But I have a 30-year history that tells me it's just not going to be that way. How long would it take me to lose this weight? Sixty years, maybe. Well, it comes down to this: I'm either going to get on with it and live my life today, or I'm going to stop, hang up on life, and that's the end of it.

One of the things I noticed was when I put an end to the conversation, so did everybody else.

Glenda: That inner voice is very sneaky—you have to be vigilant and continue to catch it. After a while, you know it's there, but you don't give it too much credibility. I mean, when you really think about it, that voice is an uninvited pest! It's like a mild but nagging stiff neck that has to be exercised out.

Gail: What about clothes? Did you make any changes in the way you were dressing?

Leah: I'm dressing better now. I buy and wear beautiful silks, which I wouldn't have done before—I was into polyester, whatever was cheap. I don't wait anymore until I can fit into a size 10 to buy myself something pretty. And what's wonderful is that we have all these great shops for larger-size women now. (Dangerous, too—but wonderful!)

Joanne: I threw everything out of the closet that was too small. Afterward, I knew that every time I pulled something off a hanger, it would fit me. Then I started buying clothes for myself. Normally, when you feel fat, you wear a lot of black. I was buying yellows, more vital, brighter colors and styles I never would have worn, like full skirts with wide belts. I didn't gain any more weight, and I had sanity!

Carolyn: My wardrobe has changed because more fashionable clothes are available to me. When I first went back to work full-time in 1974, I had to buy what the magazine, *Big Beautiful Woman*, calls bullet-proof polyester—black, navy, and blue clothes. Now I definitely wear more colorful clothes that I love and that complement my skin—purples, lavenders, and hot pinks. Who knows, I may even start wearing fringed sweaters now.

Carol: I've always hated clothes shopping, not because I can't find anything that I like, just because I just don't like shopping! But now I notice that when I do shop, I'm buying colors that "fit" me better. Rather than the blacks and dark, somber colors, I've now got bright blues, whites, peaches, and greens. And I'm trying different styles. I'm just much more comfortable with whatever I've got on, so I don't worry about what I'm wearing.

Sue: There isn't anything worse on Earth than waking up with that interior conversation that begins, "God, I'm a fat slob!" And then you look in your closet and none of your outfits are a size 10—or even worse, they're all a size too small! It's really awful to keep clothes in your closet that don't fit you. I mean, that's an *insane* action—insane, as in completely unhealthy!

I've got a closet full of clothes. I spend money! And I'm extremely picky; I've been coached by a brilliant consultant who specializes in large-size women and is absolutely the best! I know all the good and bad large-size dress shops in my city; I know the price ranges, the clothes they carry, all of it! I never do what fat people normally do. They say, "I'll buy something next week after I lose 5 pounds—that will be my reward." You know what happens to them in that week? They *gain* 10 pounds! You can't put it off until you lose weight. You have to think about how many years it's been since you've lost weight.

Glenda: People who think they're fat always have a lot of shoes, jackets, and scarves, and one or two "uniforms"—usually in black. Well, I've stopped looking at shoe windows as much. Now I'm looking at real clothes! I'm wearing dresses in reds and blues with belts and peplums. I've found that by not weighing myself, I don't put as many restrictions on what I can wear. The last time I went shopping, I realized I had actually dropped two dress sizes! Was I excited? Sure! I never dreamed that weight would fall off me without a lot of agony—but it did, it really did!

Gail: What about self-nurturance? Did you introduce any new personal touches into your life?

Joanne: I'm still learning to nurture myself in other ways. To me, food was always Mommy. My own mother was always feeding me and then when I was 6, my parents divorced and she left me. I had a big abandonment issue and food became my missing mom. That's how I nurtured myself. What else could I do besides give myself food? What other treats? Well, I started to learn.

I discovered massage—it's wonderful! And my makeup. I changed it, even had my eyebrows reshaped! I began to take good care of my hair. But even more significant for me was having beautiful, long nails for the first time in my life! I started having manicures and getting tips and wraps. When I paid more attention to myself, I felt better about myself. And I joined a health club for the first time in my life, even though I was uncomfortable at first, being the only heavy person there. It's interesting that even now when I don't feel totally comfortable with myself and start obsessing, I exercise. But I try to use my treadmill at least four times a week—obsessing or not. It's a good habit I've acquired.

Sue: Every time I walk out of my house, I want to know that my presentation to the world is complete and that I look great. I'm very, very sensitive in terms of how I put myself together. If I have to walk into a staff meeting and I'm not ready for it—physically prepared—my attention won't be on the business that needs to be done.

Glenda: The best thing I did for myself was to join a gym. I've been going to a low-impact aerobics class about three times a week. If I'm too tired to do the workout, I start slowly, using the equipment. After a while, my body wakes up and I'll join the class. You know, everything you've read about exercise being a great mood elevator is true. I feel like a different person when I walk out of the gym.

Gail: A lot of women have talked about gaining a new sense of confidence and heightened self-esteem. Has the program helped you in this area?

Carolyn: Yes. For years and years I wanted to be one of the lay readers at church, but I had decided I was too fat! "I'll do that when I'm thinner," I thought. Now, still at the same weight, I'm speaking before very large groups of people. It's an incredible change! And I also started giving workshops on the subject of time management and self-esteem! It's not as if you totally forget about your weight—I still have to catch myself when I start drifting into weight worries.

Sometimes I think: "Are these people wondering how I could be giving them good advice when I'm so heavy?" But I now know that as long as I'm not thinking that way, they won't think that way. They accept me as an authority.

There's a woman about my size and weight where I work who dresses very nicely, is very attractive, and is extremely well thought of in the division. Every time I kind of get down on myself because of my size, I think of her and how much people like her. When I can't make myself believe the truth about myself, I can see the truth about her. And if it's true about her, then it appears that it's true about me as well. It's all pretty amazing!

You know, since I went to that seminar, I'm probably less concerned about how my body looks than the average woman—and I'm talking about the average woman who weighs 135! They all seem to be obsessed with their bodies and their weight.

Carol: One of the major benefits of the program was that it helped me develop a lot more self-confidence. You just forget about the weight. It isn't your be-all or end-all. One thing the program did for me was to teach me to say, "Hey, you're you! What you are inside and how you react to people—not the body image!" And I think it just helped me focus on the internal person rather than the external.

The image idea hasn't entirely vanished, but I don't worry about it because I'm more caught up in the relationships I've developed. I meet people more easily now—as equals. And I'm accepted more easily. When you have confidence in yourself, people accept you for what you are.

Leah: I work at an office job during the day and I've also been singing professionally for years and years. And I'm singing better than ever now. At auditions, I not only want them to hear my singing, I want them to see my personality. I've also started studying improvisation and that's so exciting! I'm just having a great time.

Glenda: When you get the weight obsession behind you, it's almost as if you've cleared a path for your natural self-esteem to rise. When I'm not worried about weight, I feel very powerful and competent. And those feelings just automatically give you the confidence to take new risks.

Gail: In terms of your work life, did anything change?

Leah: I've been doing all sorts of wonderful career things. After the seminar, I started buying *Backstage* and auditioning again. On my first audition, I got the part. And then I auditioned for another touring company and was doing shows and getting paid. It's just been rolling along from there. I got my first major regional contract last year, and this spring I have five different performances coming up. I do a lot of cabaret work and last year I did a one-woman show three times. It's very exciting. I know that all of this started after the seminar—I was ready to audition again.

Sue: I've never let my weight interfere with my sense of authority. I'm not sure why. When I was a manager of a division, I would sit in on meetings with all the other managers, mostly men. It just never bothered me—it doesn't exist in my realm of reality. I'm still very overweight and it's not the way I prefer to be, but I'm not that involved with how other people perceive me.

Since I'm no longer concerned with what people think about my body, they think what I want them to think! There are a lot of people I've bumped into in my life who have an "attitude" about weight, but I have to tell you, it's been a long time since I've come up against anybody like that.

I interviewed for a job several years ago when I probably weighed about 275, and it was a really important interview for me. I would be working for a space program, a job I really wanted. During the interview, the man who was asking the questions said, "You know, I don't mean to be personal, but I really run around in that building and I need you to be able to keep up with me." Then he asked, "Is your weight going to hamper you?" I answered, "Well, I don't think so. I can't imagine that it would—it never has before." That was all he said, and then he hired me.

Interestingly, I knew I was up against one other person and, whoever it was, I figured that the person I had beat out must have been a real dope. Then about a year later, I found out she was an executive director and looked like a starlet—slim, dark brown curly hair to her shoulders, wore leather pants. I couldn't believe it.

Carolyn: I'm an administrative officer in a government research lab. I manage about a $45-million research budget. Since the seminar, my division nominated me for an annual award for contributions and I won it! My family attended the ceremony and I made a speech that really went over well. Then I won another award—it's been, God, just really great!

During the seminar, Steve said some incredible things to me about how powerful I was. All my life, I had been trying to ignore that sense of power because girls of my generation were socialized to think that we weren't supposed to be very strong. We were supposed to be meek and passive; if we were powerful, we had better hide it quickly before we were caught by someone! That was sort of the way I had lived my life. If I caught myself doing anything too powerful, well, I just squelched it fast. But in spite of my best efforts—it still kept coming out! I kept being successful in things that I did! At the seminar, I felt I was in a safe place and it was okay to find out more.

I will never forget Steve's telling me, "I can't imagine what you could have done with your life if you hadn't spent all that energy on dieting and working so hard to keep your weight under control." It was an absolutely mind-boggling thought! And such a loud and clear message to me.

Carol: I have always been the type of person who went ahead and did what she felt like doing. But since the seminar, I'm even more so. I just can't emphasize enough the confidence it gave me! I've always been a friendly, gregarious person, but I didn't have the confidence I have now! Especially when it comes to meeting new people.

My job entails talking to directors of divisions and finding out what they need. I just got back from an out-of-town conference with over 5,000 people. When I'd start up a conversation, it was fascinating to see the way the people reacted to me. You know, I don't think I would have done that before I attended the seminar—especially with men. I was somewhat timid then and I held back because I didn't know how I would be accepted—I stayed in the background. But on this last trip, we were all just relaxed and comfortable, easily conversing, going to dinner, happy with each other's company.

Now that I don't worry about my weight and it's no longer my preoccupation, I have more success with people in my job. And it goes across the board with everyone, no matter what their age or position.

Gail: Has your general health changed?

Sue: My health is 9,000 times better than it was. For me, the nutritional information was the single most important aspect of the seminar. I'm sensitive to a lot of foods. And my immune system has been kind of beaten up, which causes a lot of different problems. When I went to the seminar, I found out about foods I could eat that didn't cause reactions and foods that definitely helped my health. I didn't have to restrict my foods—I could actually choose foods that were good for me and tasted good. I definitely stopped being sick as much with congestion, colds, and allergy reactions.

Carol: Before I started the seminar, I had gone through a period of severe headaches and dizziness. I had had a glucose tolerance test that showed that I was borderline diabetic. I also had a high blood pressure problem. My doctor had me on medication and told me point blank, "You have to lose at least 125 pounds before you're going to come to grips with any of these problems."

A month or two after I went to the seminar, I realized I felt much better. My blood pressure had normalized to the point at which I told my doctor I wanted to go off the medication for a weekend to see what would happen. I took none of the medication from that Friday until the next Tuesday. On the following Friday, I had my blood pressure checked. It was normal! It was checked again on Monday. It was still normal. My doctor took me off the medication. She was amazed. "I don't know how you did it without the medication," she said, "but there's no need to take it anymore." At this point, I asked for another glucose tolerance test. It also came back completely normal! This is for real.

It took about two months. I just changed my eating habits in accordance with the Body-Signal Program. Recently, I went to another one of my doctors and had a new series of blood tests done. He said, "I don't how you're doing it, but keep it up. I wish every patient who walked in this office could have a blood work report like this." Everything was completely normal. The cholesterol levels, the triglycerides, the sugar levels—everything! My blood pressure is still a little high, but we *were* talking 180 over 110, now we're talking 140 over 74.

Gail: What about intimate relationships with men?

Joanne: Well, my boyfriend thinks I'm terrific. As for me, I know that when I feel good about myself, I also feel more sensual.

I learned something else that's very important: If I eat sugar—at least too much of it—it kills my sexual urges, and when I go to bed, I just want to go to sleep.

Sue: When I stopped concentrating on my appearance, so did everybody else. And my husband is absolutely thrilled. I met him when I was over 200 pounds. He has a wonderful body—very fit and trim. He works out every day, runs marathons, and does triathlons. And we have a wonderful sex life. But I remember times in the past when we'd be walking somewhere and I'd turn to him and say, "Look, you've got to feel conspicuous walking with a woman my size. Forget that I'm you're wife for a minute. Don't you feel the least bit embarrassed?" And he'd look at me and say, "I really don't, honest to God. But I can work at it if you want me to."

How you choose to feel about relationships with men depends on how you really want to live your life. If you want to live single and alone, then avoid meeting men from fear of rejection as some heavy women do. I promise you— that fear will keep you single.

Leah: I'm divorced. I don't think I've intentionally put men on hold. I haven't really met anybody I want to get involved with—but then, I haven't been looking for anybody either. I don't give it a lot of thought right now, probably because I don't feel a lack. I've been too busy with my life to be on the lookout for a man. But I'm ready to meet the right one.

Carol: I'm a widow and not interested in getting involved with anyone right now. But because of my new confidence, I can now look on men as friends. And that does change things.

Glenda: I know there are men out there who are attracted only to thin, slender, reedlike women. But then I know there are a lot of other men—a *lot* of them—who don't use that as a criterion. I've been divorced for about ten years, and during that time I went out with a lot of different men.

For the past two years, I've been involved with a man who thinks I'm divine! I've been aware of something interesting in this relationship. When I used to get into my weight-worry slumps and hate myself, I'd very subtly avoid him and he'd move away from me. But when I feel good about myself, he picks up on that energy and he's right there! He says the self-loathing confuses him. I understand why.

Gail: You've got the floor totally right now. What advice do you want to give to other women?

Leah: Diets don't work! If I've learned one thing, it's this: The less you eat, the less food your body gets accustomed to eating and you can end up gaining weight on 1,200 calories a day. Love yourself as you are! Don't wait until you're the ideal size to do what you want to do. Your size has nothing to do with being successful and getting what you want from life. You're okay just as you are. Self-acceptance is everything.

Joanne: Do whatever it takes to learn to love and accept yourself. It's so sad, so criminal, to torment and torture yourself about your weight your whole life. I know it's hard to let go of the obsession, but unless you do, your life is over already! When you're in a lot of pain, you may want to smother it with food. But if you stay aware of your worth, are vigilant against defeatism, and get your feelings out into the open, you won't need to act them out by stuffing yourself.

Sue: If you've gone from a size 10 to a 16, throw out all the 10's and buy only 16's! You should have a closet full of size 16's that are absolutely smashing! I'm sometimes stunned at the way some of my heavy friends treat themselves. I say to them, "Please, don't go out of the house looking like that! Put some lipstick on—comb your hair. I don't care if you're 2 hours late. Make a phone call and say you broke your foot. Wrap it in a bandage if you have to, but go in there looking fantastic!" When you hate yourself, it opens the door to gaining weight.

Carol: Acceptance works. I am satisfied with myself. And that satisfaction gives off a strong sense of confidence that allows me to interact with other people as equals, as real colleagues and friends.

Glenda: Stop depriving yourself of food, stop treating your body like an enemy, and stop treating yourself like an outsider! You and your body count! When you accept yourself, you no longer want to be invisible and you no longer apologize for taking up too much space. That attitude is so abusive—and it's a lie! When you start listening to your Body Signals and the momentum gets going, you start believing the truth.

Carolyn: Believe it! The whole Body-Signal concept is so worth-while. The fat is in your head! This isn't a gimmick—it's real!

Chapter 9

Your Body Signals: The Can't-Miss Guide to Becoming an Instinctive Eater

You must eat whenever you're hungry— and stop as soon as you're satisfied.

You're now going to learn the secret that only 4½ billion people know: how to respond to your Body Signals and become an Instinctive Eater. By the time you reach the end of this chapter, you'll understand the distinction between what *you* want and what your *body* wants. In the beginning, your understanding will be somewhat intellectual, but as you continue practicing these skills, the distinction will be gradually internalized. If you're overweight, it won't be long before you'll begin to shed those excess pounds and reach your optimal weight.

Beginners, Spinners, and Super-Spinners

People have achieved different levels of expertise in their chosen fields. For example, I'm a virtuoso Instinctive Eater totally in tune with my Body Signals. Right behind me are people who are beginners, and in back of that group are the people who are aware something's off with their skills, but don't know what to do to become experts. I call these people spinners. Trailing the spinners are the super-spinners, the people who can be likened to "a bull in a china shop"—more to the point, to *dieters.* They still don't realize something's wrong with what they're doing, even though they continue to crash into walls over and over again.

How do you stop the "spin" or the "super-spin"? By learning to tune in to your Body Signals and becoming a beginning Instinctive Eater. I can already hear your objections: You want to become a virtuoso right away. You'd like to be able to eat whatever you want, whenever you want, without conscious thought. But it's too early.

For now, just imagine what it would be like if you were about to become a swimmer and were beginning at the spinner stage. You don't know how to swim, but you do know that there's something you need to learn. Okay. You're sitting in my class, and I'm giving you a chalk talk on how to become a swimmer. I tell you how to move your arms and your head, and how to breathe correctly. And now I throw you into the deep end. Not feeling too confident about your ability to stay afloat, right? Don't be disheartened. You're not confident because you're still a spinner: You're not yet a beginning swimmer.

But what if I give you the experience of being a swimmer? What if I place you in the shallow end of the pool, instruct you to hold on to the sides while I demonstrate all the strokes, and then ask you to paddle around in the shallow end? This time, when I throw you into the deep end, you'll actually swim around a bit.

Feels different, doesn't it? Your confidence is greater because you're now a beginning swimmer. You're no longer frightened of swimming pools—you have a new relationship with the water. Even better, you know you can swim. (You could, if you wanted, become a virtuoso Olympic swimmer. That's entirely up to you.) But for now, swimming itself is no problem.

That's exactly how you're going to learn to become a beginning Instinctive Eater and respond to your Body Signals. You're going to accustom yourself to food, and as a result, you'll be able to handle it anytime, anywhere, confident that there will be no problem.

Let's face it. You're lucky that I'm not teaching you to swim, because if I were, I couldn't guarantee 100 percent success. Fortunately, I am teaching you a skill that I know you can learn—that everyone can learn. Many of you are shaking your heads just now, silently and skeptically asking, "If I've been an Overeater all my life and am unaware of my Body Signals, how can he say with 100 percent certainty that he can teach me to become an Instinctive Eater and honor my Body Signals?"

The answer bears repeating: If you were already in touch with your Body Signals and for some oddball reason asked: "Could you please teach me how to lose them?" I couldn't do it. You'd be asking me to teach you to move from a natural to an unnatural state. It just wouldn't work. But we're talking about teaching a natural skill—how to do what's *instinctive*. The learning will be automatic. That's why I guarantee you 100 percent success. One hundred percent of the people who want to learn how to become Instinctive Eaters inevitably do.

How You Lost Your Body Signals

It began with dieting—or deprivation. (At this point, you're well aware that they're synonymous.) Let's flash backward for a moment and recall a time when you decided to go on a diet. Right off, you began to deny yourself food. In short order, you experienced hunger. You tried to ignore the hunger, which means that you had to ignore your Body Signals. What was the upshot? Eventually, you lost touch with them. They stopped making themselves known, and if they did emerge, you couldn't recognize them. That's precisely what happened to many of you dieters.

When you let yourself become too hungry, a natural response occurs. You binge! You don't binge because you're crazy, because you're cursed with a psychological defect, or because deep down in your subconscious you hate your mother and want to wreak revenge on her for what she did to you when you were 3 years old. You binge simply because *you dieted and went too long without eating!* And again, what does it mean to binge? It means you eat and eat and eat some more. It means that you run roughshod over your Satisfaction Signal and lose touch with it.

Now you're really in trouble! Your Hunger Signals and your Satisfaction Signals have disappeared! How can you possibly know what to do around food? How can you possibly know when to eat, what to eat, how to eat? The answer, of course: You don't know!

Stress and Bingeing

At this point, you can't distinguish hunger, and you can't distinguish satisfaction. What's left? Eating in response to external cues—other people's schedules (my husband/wife is eating, so I guess I'll eat, too), the numbers on the clock (it's 6:00 P.M., time for dinner), business schedules (in my office, lunch is between 1:00 and 2:00), and eating in response to emotions, which is only natural. After all, you're on a diet, and a diet is about as stressful a self-imposed torture as you can diabolically conceive.

Now consider this: While you're on this diet, your boss tells you that your work is below par and if you don't shape up, you're going to be out of a job in two weeks. The stress cords tighten. What do you do about it? Simple. You stick your head in the refrigerator and start bingeing.

It doesn't take too long before bingeing becomes associated with stress. After a few more stressful events like the run-in with your boss, you begin to pair diet with stress, then bingeing with stress. Quite soon, dieting itself becomes secondary. Just experience some unexpected stress and you'll start bingeing. Your mate or lover says he's thinking of leaving you, and before you can murmur, "I think we should talk," your head's in the refrigerator and you don't even know how it got there! It's normal.

As a result of dieting, that's what happens. Diets foster hunger. Hunger promotes stress. Stress leads to bingeing. Given the continual stress you experience from dieting, soon you can't distinguish between hunger and boredom, hunger and fear, hunger and loneliness, hunger and anxiety—and sometimes you can't even tell the difference between hunger and thirst! Your Body Signals have gone underground.

There is no equivocation in this statement: *Until you relearn your Body Signals, you have no shot at obtaining your optimal weight*—that stable weight you're going to remain at for the rest of your life.

Let me take a moment to offer a personal confession. If I went on a diet, you can bet that I would binge. As a matter of fact, even though I never diet, I *do* binge. On the days when I've scheduled myself poorly and have had to see patients on my lunch break, or when I've worked late at the office and have gone 2 hours past the time I wanted to eat, when I get around food—I explode into it! My responses are exactly like yours. It's natural. Further, I'll explode into whatever food is put in front of me—cakes, pies, cookies. When I've gone too long without eating, I binge.

So, how do we get around this dilemma?

The Diet/Hunger Band

For the purposes of our training, let's make a diet analogous to a rubber band. Picture this: One end of the rubber band is looped around one hand. Your other hand is pulling on the band.

Now imagine this scenario. You wake up at 9:00 A.M. and you're hungry. The diet band stretches. At 10:00, you're a little hungrier and the band stretches further. At 11:00, you're more than a little hungry, but holding out—and that band is becoming taut. Noon arrives and you're close to starving, but your lunch hour doesn't begin for an hour. When 1:00 arrives and the food is placed in front of you, that band is stretched to the max, you let go with a snap, and boom! You explode into the food. You don't eat it; you blast into it! That's what dieting does for you. That's what hunger creates.

Picture yourself reenacting this same scene repeatedly over the course of your lifetime! Say at age 11, your mom and your doctor decided to put you on your first diet. During that diet, you accumulated x amount of hunger. By age 20, you've been on 10 more diets. Now you've accumulated $10x$ amount of hunger. By age 30, you've amassed the hunger from 15 more diets; at 40 the hunger is still building; and as you become older, you continue to add on more and more. Over the course of your lifetime, you accumulate so much hunger that you find that when you're not "white knuckling" it through diets and hunger, you're blasting into food! Your whole life reverberates between deprivation and explosive attacks on refrigerators and plates.

The Hunger Scale

Now picture a hunger scale from 1 to 10. It would look like this.

1	5	10
Extreme hunger	Satisfaction (the "perfect" meal)	Extreme overeating

At 1, you're so hungry, if you don't eat within the next 2 minutes, it's a sure thing that you're going to pass out. You're also sure that if you see someone with food in hand, you'll kill for it. Picture the 1 situation in your mind. Recall that experience. Your hunger is so severe, you'd steal food from a child. Feel what you felt. See what you saw. Hear what you heard. If you cannot remember being at a 1, make it up. What words would you use to describe that experience: fear, anxiety, panic, emptiness, greed, pain?

That's what severe hunger feels like. It's analogous to dieting.

Now let's move to the other extreme, a 10. You've just eaten the equivalent of four Thanksgiving dinners. You not only can't move, you're about to burst. You've placed an emergency phone call to the nearest construction company to deliver a crane—you need to be hauled from the table. Gravity has taken on a new and alarming meaning—food is rising back up through your esophagus. (You've actually eaten that much!) Picture the 10 situation. And again, feel what you felt, see what you saw, hear what you heard. Step back into that scene. Re-experience it. What words would you use to describe the experience: awful, disgusting, nauseating, painful, sick, out of control?

That's what extreme overeating feels like. And it's analogous to bingeing.

Now let's try the experience of an Instinctive Eater. Imagine the perfect meal—a 5. Picture yourself at home or at a lovely restaurant, perhaps in a country setting. Feel the way you felt. If you can't remember actually experiencing a 5, make it up. In your mind's eye, live out a time when you had the perfect meal. You might have to send yourself back to the age of 5 or 15. It doesn't matter. At this meal, you ate just the right amount; you felt pleasantly satisfied. And you ate only the foods that you genuinely enjoy, the foods that make you feel good. Again, picture that meal in your mind. Experience it. Imagine how it would feel to always eat to a 5. The 5 experience is how Instinctive Eaters eat. And this is exactly how all of your meals are going to be handled.

To keep the experience straight, I'd like you to become aware of something particularly interesting. From now on, as you eat your meals, notice that after you've finished the entrée, you'll probably have arrived at a 5, and that adding dessert will bring you up to a 7 or an 8.

I almost never eat dessert, yet I eat something sweet just about every day. I still have those cravings from the days when I was a junk food addict. (Back then, I used to feel that a day was not complete without a Milky Way.) Today I buy cookies and candy from the health food stores, but they contain no sugar; instead, they're sweetened with a little bit of fruit juice. To me, cookies and candy are still associated with pleasure, but now I find substitutes for the sugar craving. (We'll discuss sugar cravings later when we talk about substitutes for junk food on page 151.)

To keep the record straight, remember that Instinctive Eaters *do* overeat on occasion. Sometimes they eat to a 7 or an 8. But there's a major difference between you and them: They do it in control and out of choice. I'm a virtuoso Instinctive Eater and if you think I never pig out—think again! (If we should happen to be at the same party, you might see me scarfing up that food. I don't do it often, but when I do, it's by choice, and you can bet I savor every single bite.) As a virtuoso Instinctive Eater, I can also binge in control. But remember, you're a *beginner,* and bingeing isn't something you want to do. Just keep in mind that as you become more confident, as you become more than a beginner, on occasion, you'll binge, and you'll do it fully in control, for fun!

When you habitually respond to your Body Signals, Mother Nature provides you with a bonus. As you learned in chapter 3, noradrenalin, a hormone that increases your metabolic rate, is released into your bloodstream, ensuring that you won't gain an ounce when you binge. Unfortunately, Chronic Overeaters don't receive the same benefits of that hormone. The release of noradrenalin won't increase your metabolic rate, but it will increase your pulse rate and your blood pressure. Over many years, that negative metabolic effect can cause serious health consequences.

The Narcotic Effect of Overeating

For now, stay with the idea that you want to eat just the right amount of food. When you eat to a 7 or an 8, you can count on a negative metabolic effect. Like a successful narcotic, eating to an 8 metabolically drugs you. If you're experiencing stressful emotions—your boss is yelling at you, your husband or wife is neglecting you, your child is sick— who needs Valium? You've got food, and food will do the trick. Do you need more proof? Just eat to a 7 or an 8 and check out how you feel. The reason Instinctive Eaters don't use food as a narcotic is not only valid but critical: They care too much for themselves. They've developed more appropriate ways to deal with their emotions. When you eat to a 7 or an 8, you may temporarily lull your negative emotions, but there's still one emotional aftereffect that Overeaters can count on: guilt.

Eat When You're Hungry!

It sounds simplistic, but it's critical to becoming an Instinctive Eater. *You must eat when you're hungry!* I have a special theory about hunger. It goes like this. Mother Nature knows what she wants. She gave us

Body Signals for a reason: The Hunger Signal is a call for fuel. If you eat when you're hungry, you provide your body with the fuel it needs to function properly. You don't have to worry—it won't convert the food into excess fat. Conversely, when Mother Nature is not calling for food, and you eat even though you're not hungry, or you eat past satisfaction, your body doesn't know what to do with the excess and will store it as fat. That's why eating *past* satisfaction puts on weight, while eating *to* satisfaction will allow you to reach your optimal weight.

How to Know When You're Hungry

It's crucial for you to learn how to know when your body is hungry. When you're too hungry or too tired, you make wrong choices. (Having lost touch with your Body Signals, you probably haven't made too many right choices about food for a long time.) At the outset, you want to determine whether your body is hungry or your emotions are hungry. To make that determination, try to locate your Hunger Signal by searching out *where* you experience hunger, and then, *how* you experience it.

To locate the hunger in your body, try to pinpoint where the hunger is coming from. Is it in your stomach? If it is, what does it feel like? Is it a gnawing, a pain, a growling, a grumbling, an ache, bloating, or a feeling of emptiness? Is the hunger located in your chest? Do you feel a pain or a pressure? Maybe the hunger is signaling you from your head. Do you have a headache, slight dizziness, a little light-headedness, a feeling of weakness? Is the hunger cuing you from one of these areas? Is there one sensation, or several?

Look for your Hunger Signal every day. When you spot it, feed yourself and determine whether or not your body feels right. If you practice this skill daily, very soon you'll be eating only in response to true hunger.

For now, however, you need to begin to get in touch with these experiences and find out how your particular Hunger Signal manifests itself. You may not be able to locate the hunger immediately. Remember, you're practicing a new skill. If I had just explained how to do a jackknife dive into the water, do you think you could go directly to the pool and make a perfect dive? The answer, of course, is no. As with swimming, you have to practice this skill every day until it's developed.

Tomorrow morning when you wake up, don't panic. Just wait. As you go through your day, ask yourself: "Is my body sending me a Hunger Signal?" If you think the answer is yes, then eat and enjoy it. And if the answer is no, then don't eat. If you wake up tomorrow at 6:00 A.M., go through the day as usual, and still haven't picked up any Hunger Signals, don't eat! Believe me, your body won't let you starve to death. Eventually, you will reconnect with your Hunger Signals. This is a skill that must be practiced.

How Often Can You Eat?

How often do Instinctive Eaters eat? As often as they're hungry. Maybe five or six times a day. They never let themselves go hungry and deprive their body of fuel. As you'll discover (if you're now eating in response to your emotions), when you start nurturing your body and responding to its signals, and when you begin to satisfy yourself with food appropriately, you'll lose the impulse to eat the seventh, eighth, or ninth time. You'll begin to avoid putting food into your mouth until you feel the Hunger Signal—even if that means going 12 hours or a full day without eating. You won't feel deprived.

I eat about five or six times a day. After awakening, before eating breakfast, I wait until I feel the Hunger Signal. Sometimes I'm hungry immediately. Sometimes I'm not. If no Hunger Signal emerges, I take food to work with me and arrange time between patients to take care of myself. If it's a very busy day with one patient after the other, and hunger signals me—believe it, I stop and eat! I figure it's better to focus on the patient's problem than on my hunger.

What do I eat? Whole-grain muffins with no sugar that I purchase at health food stores. Sometimes I eat brown rice crackers with a little almond butter. I also eat sandwiches made with whole-grain bread and apple butter. You can make your sandwiches with whatever appeals to you—tuna, chicken, chicken salad—anything you want. The key here is to avoid sugar and white flour products (see chapter 11).

I usually begin to feel hunger again around noon, and then again when I finish seeing patients in the afternoon. At that point, I might eat a piece of fruit—a bunch of grapes, an apple, a plum. Sometimes I eat those terrific cookies sweetened with fruit juice from the health food stores or a piece of naturally sweetened carrot cake. A few hours later, I usually find myself getting hungry for dinner. In the early evening, I'm often hungry again, so I might eat another piece of fruit, some more cookies, popcorn, or whole wheat pretzels. If I'm thirsty, I drink bottled water or seltzer, sometimes sweetened with a little fruit juice.

I eat as often as I'm hungry!

How to Eat on Off-Hours

Again, as an Overeater, you don't eat when your body is hungry—and you must! Unlike an Instinctive Eater, an Overeater will give you all the reasons why she can't eat when she's hungry. "My schedule is too busy . . . The meeting ran 2 hours past lunch . . . My family eats at a certain time . . . I work for a company that designates noon as the lunch hour." Instinctive Eaters are baffled by these ideas.

Here's what you do. You eat when you're hungry, you stop when you're satisfied. It's easier than you think. Take a sandwich, a muffin, rice cakes, or fruit to work with you and keep your food handy in a desk drawer. If you're at a 2-hour meeting and your Hunger Signal has put you on alert, simply say, "Why don't we take a 10-minute restroom break?" With that, you rush back to your office, grab the snack you stashed in your drawer, and eat (see chapter 5).

Remember, if your Hunger Signal emerges five or six times a day, those cues will occur fairly close to lunchtime and to dinnertime. Don't worry about lunch and don't worry about dinner. Don't make problems where none exist. That's an Overeater's characteristic. If it's noontime and you're not hungry, don't eat. Sit with your friends or colleagues and enjoy the conversation. If it's dinnertime and you're perfectly satisfied, when your family sits down to eat, sit down with them! (Most often, they just want your company and don't care whether you eat with them or not.) Of course, if you're an Overeater, here's the first worry that will strike you: But how can I deprive myself by just sitting there when everyone else is eating! The answer is simple: If you're hungry for food, eat! But if you're satisfied, you won't experience deprivation. Eating when you're not hungry means you're eating to satisfy an emotion!

You now know how to eat during off-hours. You're going to eat in response to hunger—*whenever you're hungry!* Once your body has stabilized and is accustomed to the fact that you're listening to it and respecting its cues, you'll probably experience a Hunger Signal approximately every 3 hours.

Many years ago, at the time my first Lighten Up seminar was held, participants were allowed to eat only at the meal breaks. Not wanting to be labeled a hypocrite, I also waited for the designated eating time. Although I was teaching a group of people who weren't tuned in to their Body Signals, I was (and still am) extremely sensitive to mine. I remember waiting for the break, growing hungrier and hungrier, completely ignoring my Body Signals. When meal breaks finally arrived, I'd walk into a restaurant and explode into my food. I wound up sick from overeating. Since I was the one teaching the seminar, the situation was rather embarrassing! Fortunately, the following time slot was run by my partner—there was no way I could even consider resuming the seminar for the next hour. (I've changed the rules at Lighten Up since then. For the two seminar days *only,* I now define an Instinctive Eater as a person who eats when *I'm* hungry!)

How to Know When You're Satisfied

The definition of *satiety* is the absence of hunger or the point of satisfaction. They both mean the same thing. When you're a beginning Instinctive Eater learning your Body Signals, you decide if you're satisfied by continually asking yourself this question: "Am I still hungry?" It's critical to remember that if you began eating when you weren't hungry, there's little chance of recognizing the absence of hunger.

Most of us are familiar with this experience: In the middle of dinner, the phone rings. You stop eating, run to answer it, and even though you tell the person that you'll call them back, the caller insists on telling you "just one thing." By the time you get back to the table, *you're no longer hungry!* While you were running to the phone, talking to the friend, and returning to the table, you had stopped eating and your body had a chance to decide whether or not it was satisfied. Had there been no interruption, you might have eaten to a 7 or an 8. Remember, it often takes 15 to 20 minutes for your body to register the Satisfaction Signal. Stay alert for the signal from your stomach to your brain, and when you get it, push your plate away.

The Satisfaction Signal, like the Hunger Signal, needs to be relearned. During my seminars, many participants have talked about how they perceived the Satisfaction Signal but chose to neglect it in favor of the food in front of them. For this particular group, the signal didn't totally elude them—they simply denied it.

I liken the experience to that of many of my elderly patients whose bowels no longer move and want prescribed laxatives. The analogy works. For much of their lives, they ignored the body's elimination signal. Why? They were "too busy." Eventually, they lost the function.

That's what happens when you ignore your Hunger Signals and your Satisfaction Signals. Fortunately, these signals can be relearned.

How Long Will It Take to Relearn Your Body Signals?

My most resistant student was a woman who, essentially, had been on a diet for 35 years. It took her six months to relearn her Body Signals. After the seminar, she called me several times.

"I don't think your system is working for me," she said.

"Why not?" I asked.

"I still don't know when I'm hungry, and I haven't lost any weight," she answered.

Her calls went on for months. One day she phoned and said, "It's still not working."

"Why not?" I asked again.

"Well," she said, "I'm still not sure when I'm hungry."

I needed to know more. "Have you practiced what I taught you about locating your Hunger Signals?" I asked.

She was adamant. "I practice it every day!"

"Why don't you think it's working?" I asked again.

"Because I still haven't lost any weight," she told me.

"Okay," I said. "How many times have you binged in the last month?"

She thought about it, then finally answered, "Once."

"What did you binge on?" I asked.

"I had a slice of bread," she said, "and I wasn't hungry for it."

"And you're telling me that you haven't gotten results from the Lighten Up seminar?" I exclaimed. "Just hang in there." Six months from the date of her seminar, she called me again and said: "I now know when I'm hungry, and my body is shrinking. It took six months, but my blouse size went from a size 42 to a size 14." That woman now knows when she's hungry and eats, and she knows when she's satisfied and stops.

Much like developing breath control while swimming, learning this skill takes practice. Your body may need a little time to catch on to the fact that you're caring for it again—it has an intelligence of its own. If you've done nothing but abuse it for years through dieting and bingeing, that intelligence is suspicious. It needs some time to catch up. Your body may not trust your new habits until it knows you mean business. Remember, relearning your Body Signals is not the same as dieting. It's not a quick fix. It may take time, but it's worth it.

How to Eat What You Really Want

Now that you've learned to locate where your hunger is coming from and you've begun to learn how to experience it, you'll need to know if you're eating the foods that you really want. How do you know?

Virtuoso Instinctive Eaters know *naturally* what they want to eat.

But as a beginning Instinctive Eater, you must relearn your authentic desires and remain extremely alert.

Ask yourself the following questions.

- What taste do I want—sweet, sour, bitter, or spicy?
- What temperature do I want—hot, cold, or room temperature?
- What consistency do I want—a food like pudding, steak, or something else?
- What texture do I want—crunchy, soft, chewy, or smooth?
- Do I want liquid or solid, wet or dry, soft or hard?

Go through the checklist. The more questions you ask, the better chance you'll have of eating exactly what your body wants. For now, if you feel like you want to eat pizza or a bacon cheeseburger, go ahead and eat it.

But you must remember to ask yourself, "Did I want this food before I saw it?" And, "Is my body hungry?" If the answer is yes on both counts, enjoy it. If the answer is no, back off.

How to Handle Sugar Cravings

There is one caveat to eating what you want. Many times you will confuse your Hunger Signal with sugar cravings (see chapter 11). It happens to me. There's a little shop a half block from where I live that sells Italian ices, cakes, and pastries. Often, when I find myself walking by that shop, I notice I crave everything in the window. It takes a moment for me to realize what's actually occurring: I'm hungry. If I eat some broiled fish and broccoli sautéed with a little garlic and oil, I'm satisfied. For this reason, although you've been instructed to eat whatever you want, if what you want is made with sugar, try substituting real food.

Sometimes it may turn out that sugar *is* what you really want. For example, this past summer, I was thinking a lot about Breyer's chocolate ice cream, a treat I used to eat by the gallon when I was a kid and a junk food addict. (In truth, I was 30 years old!) While making rounds at the hospital one day, covering for a vacationing colleague, I asked a patient of his, "Is there anything I can do to help make you feel better?"

"Yeah," he said. "Can you bring me in some Breyer's chocolate ice cream?"

I responded instantly. "Brother," I said, "you have yourself a soulmate."

The next day when I made my rounds, I showed up in his room with the goods: He ate his half and I ate mine.

Just recently, I was thinking about that ice cream again. I kept telling myself, "No, you're not really hungry for ice cream—it's only a sugar craving." After experiencing that same inner dialogue for a couple of days, it finally hit me—It's Breyer's chocolate ice cream that I want! I went to the deli, bought it, ate it, and reveled in every single bite. (Don't forget—I'm a virtuoso Instinctive Eater. I suggest that you don't engage in this recreational eating until you have your Body Signals down pat.)

Food Minefields

Your task is to try to make the distinction between the foods that your body really wants and the foods that just "call out" to you. You know what I mean. You're walking down the street past the food minefields of your city. The souvlaki fast food restaurants, the fresh bagel stores, the ice cream specialty shops, the popcorn concessions, fast food joints, pizza parlors, and particularly the bakeries—you know, those insidious little shops that have special blowers installed to waft the smell right out onto the street. That smell is like a hook: It reaches up into your nose and drags you into the bakery. Your eyes have already moved across the window, spotted the pastries, and landed on that one éclair pointing at you—the one that's saying, "I've got your name on me!"

You must try to avoid the foods that "call out" to you. Here's a good rule for shunning them. *If you weren't thinking of that particular food before you saw it, don't eat it!* Before you go into a restaurant, look for the menu on the outside window or door and read it. If the menu isn't available until you're seated, be sure to read it thoroughly *before* you order your food or start glancing around at other people's plates. Go through your hunger checklist on page 151 and figure out what foods you authentically desire. What foods were you thinking about before you saw the menu and before you spotted the choices on someone else's plate?

Let me tell you how this actually works. While attending a class one night, I began thinking about a carton of yogurt I had in my refrigerator. On my way home in the taxi, all I could think about was that yogurt. I really wanted it! When I arrived home and opened the refrigerator, what I saw was a lemon meringue pie (my favorite from way back when I was a sugar addict) that a house guest had left as a treat for me. "Well!" I thought, "this must be a message from God!"

Instead of eating the yogurt, I ate the pie. Later, as I was getting ready for bed, the yogurt flashed through my mind. I realized I still wanted that yogurt! Back I went to the refrigerator, and down went the yogurt. It happens to me as well as to you. If I don't eat what my body really wants the first time around, I'll find some way to get to it.

The point to remember is this: When you have a choice, eat only those foods you actually thought about and wanted before you saw them.

Be Deliberately Conscious of Food

Start to think about food carefully. Be attentive to what it is you're eating. Don't shop when you're hungry. And remember to ask yourself the most important question before you put food in your mouth: "Am I hungry?" If the answer is yes, then eat and enjoy every bite. The second question you need to ask is this: "What do I want to eat?"

Staying aware around food also means treating yourself like royalty at meals. Use your best linen or placemats, the good silverware, the company crystal and china. If you like flowers, buy them fresh and arrange them in front of you on the table where you'll be eating. If you love candlelight, buy long candles and light them just before you sit down. Arrange the table as attractively as you can. From now on, you're going to treat yourself like a guest—a special one, a favorite one.

And, while you're still in the kitchen, let me point out an interesting physical precept. I call it The Law of Dishes in the Sink. Evidence demonstrates that one dirty dish spawns another, and the more dishes there are in the sink, the more they accumulate. Keep your sink clean and your dishes washed. It sounds petty and unimportant, but the more relentless you are in your new attentiveness around food, the more conscious you'll become about your Body Signals. Stay alert.

The Body-Signal Eating Guidelines

Before you get a little nervous, let me assure you that these guidelines are not just another cluster of rules like those that have kept you harnessed to diets. They have nothing to do with dieting. The guidelines were created to help you become a beginning Instinctive Eater as quickly as possible.

Although the first few have touches of behavior modification built into them, and behavior modification has about a 100 percent failure rate, I've included these particular guidelines to heighten your consciousness around food. Again, what virtuoso Instinctive Eaters do *unconsciously*, beginning Instinctive Eaters need to do *consciously*.

Guideline 1: Nothing else. This means that when you eat, you literally do nothing else to distract you. Don't watch television, listen to the radio, read newspapers or books, do your knitting, talk on the telephone, or balance your checkbook. (I've already anticipated your next question. Yes, absolutely! If you're eating with someone else, of course you can listen, speak, engage in a dialogue!)

Guideline 2: One place. This guideline was designed strictly for eating at home. Maintain one place as your eating area, the *only* area where you eat. You might choose your kitchen table or your dining room table. It makes no difference. Overeaters tend to engage frequently in unconscious eating. For instance, you may find yourself eating in front of the television, in bed, or while walking around the house deep in thought. If you train yourself to eat in one place, you'll begin to break up those unconscious eating patterns and consciously focus on your food. (Again, I've anticipated the question that follows the introduction of this guideline: "I've selected the kitchen table as my one place, but what if guests are invited for dinner? Can I join them in the dining room?" Yes. Again, the answer, of course, is yes!)

Guideline 3: Look at your food and smell it. This guideline is designed to heighten your awareness of the food on your plate. Sure, the food is right under your nose, but Overeaters rarely observe or sense the textures, colors, or smells. Take a few seconds to look at your food, to savor the smell, to enjoy the spectacle. Remember, a plate of food is not a swimming pool! It's not something that you dive into.

Guideline 4: Chew your food! This is the most important guideline in the group. (And believe it or not, it's the hardest one to follow.) Of all the concepts I teach at the Lighten Up seminars, this one requires the most concentration, the most practice, and the most willingness on your part to change.

According to one respected study, the average American eats a meal in 6½ minutes! Think about it. That means the Thanksgiving dinner someone slaved over for three days might be devoured by some guests in 6½ minutes! It's mind-boggling, but true.

There are some solid reasons for relearning to chew your food.

For one thing, when you chew—really chew—you begin to taste food again.

Another reason for chewing thoroughly is that it helps you experience food satisfaction. I have a personal theory about chewing and overeating. It's never been scientifically tested, but I believe it's true. An Overeater can eat a ton of food and experience no satisfaction, while a new Instinctive Eater can eat a small quantity and feel totally satisfied. Why? Overeaters never actually taste their food. As a result, they never experience satisfaction. Because they aren't satisfied, they continue to crave food and to eat more and more. Essentially, the habit of overeating is acquired as a compensation of quantity for quality. (As I said, this is only a theory, and when you begin to chew your food and taste it, you can judge for yourself.)

Chewing improves your digestion. Eighty to 90 percent of the patients who come to me complaining of digestive problems—chronic stomachaches, excess gas, bloating—report that after they learned to slow down and chew their food, their symptoms disappeared.

The very act of chewing slows you down at the table. For purposes of weight control, this is an essential positive consequence. When you slow down your eating, you're able to tune in to your Satisfaction Signal. Picture this scene. There's a plate of food sitting in front of you, and your body is hungry, but only for half of it. If the whole plateful is in your stomach 6½ minutes later, your body won't have had the chance to key in to its Satisfaction Signal! It may need 15 or 20 minutes to do that. By simply chewing your food, you will have saved yourself from eating double the quantity you wanted originally—*without being on a diet!*

Guideline 5: Chew empty-handed. Put your utensils down between bites. I've never met an Overeater who could learn to chew her food unless she chewed empty-handed. Visualize yourself at the dinner table. You pick up the fork, stab a piece of food, put the food in your mouth, and before you begin to chew, your fork is stabbing the next bite. The action is so fast, it blurs before your eyes. A good way to slow down is to keep utensils out of your hands while you're chewing.

Guideline 6: Leave something. There are two reasons to leave something on your plate: You'll force yourself into the habit of tuning in to your Satisfaction Signal, and you'll break the pattern of cleaning your plate.

In my seminars, I routinely take the following survey: "Who in this room is cleaning her plate to save the kids in India? How many of you are cleaning your plate to save the kids in Europe? How about the kids in Appalachia? And what about Africa? Ethiopia? China?" As a child, which kids were you told you were saving? At this point, if you're still convinced that cleaning your plate will stop the starvation anywhere in the world, continue to eat.

Guideline 7: No nudity. No, this doesn't mean you're forbidden to eat in the raw. It's just a way of reminding you about naked-calorie foods: foods that have calories but little or no nutritional value. Essentially, there are three categories: refined sugar, white flour, and alcohol (see chapter 11).

You now know the Body-Signal Secret. You know exactly what you must do to solve your weight problem: Eat when you're hungry; chew your food slowly and thoroughly; put your utensils down between bites; taste your food; and stop eating as soon as you're satisfied. This is how you're going to reach your optimal weight and stay there.

As you begin to respond to your Body Signals and respect your body, you'll also begin to lighten your harsh judgments against yourself. Relearning your Body Signals is the key to becoming an Instinctive Eater, and becoming an Instinctive Eater is the key to weight control. Both are acts of self-love. This is the secret only 4½ billion people already know.

Chapter 10

Your Body Signals and Your Health

A total commitment to nurturing yourself is a total commitment to optimal health.

There are two words in our vocabulary that are rarely (if ever) linked together in one concept. You've probably never heard them used this way. No one—not your mother, husband, doctor, or friends—ever uses them as a harmonious unit. And if they did, you'd probably think they'd gone around the bend.

Those two words are: *fat* and *healthy.*

Contrary to everything you've been taught, those two words generally *do* belong together. Here are the facts.

- Most fat people are healthy.
- No matter what you weigh (with the exception of the very fattest and the very thinnest people), if your weight is stable, you're probably healthy.
- Attempts to lose weight (other than by listening to your Body Signals and eating nutritious foods) are more likely to damage your health than improve it.

Have you got that? Okay, then let's get personal. What about you? Are you at a healthy weight?

You may not really know. You may be only guessing. You may be working with worn-out, anachronistic assumptions. So let me help you answer that question for yourself.

Height/Weight Chart Mythology

If you're using the life insurance company weight-for-height charts as a yardstick, then, like every other dieter who uses those bogus charts as a measure of "normal" health, you're focused on a deception.

You don't believe it? Okay. Then just for a moment, although those height/weight charts are totally without scientific validity, let's pretend that they are valid.

If you're willing to believe what these charts tell you, then you're willing to believe that 35 to 40 percent of Americans (to use the United States as one example) *are* overweight.

Next, let's take a look at some of the broad surveys published both in commercial magazines and by the U.S. government. Now you find that 70 to 90 percent of Americans *perceive* themselves as having a weight problem.

Okay so far? Thirty-five to 40 percent *are* overweight, and 70 to 90 percent *think* they're overweight, but aren't. Now what? By subtracting 35 to 40 percent from 70 to 90 percent, you'll find your conclusion: About half the people who think they have a weight problem—*don't.*

Bearing in mind that we're still using those deceptive insurance charts as our measure, which group do you fall into? Do you belong to the half that, according to the charts, only *feels* overweight, but isn't? Or to the half that *is* actually overweight?

Now consider this. If you're among those who only *feel* that they're overweight (which could easily be the case), think what this implies: Even if you listen to your Body Signals and even if you control your intake of fat-promoting foods, you still won't lose weight!

Okay. But what about the 35 to 40 percent who actually *are* overweight according to these spurious charts? Don't they really have serious health risks? Shouldn't *they* lose weight? The answer is no.

At the risk of being labeled repetitious, think what this implies: Even if you listen to your Body Signals and even if you control your intake of fat-promoting foods, you still won't lose weight!

The Body-Signal Contradiction

"I won't lose weight??!"

I can feel your outrage even as this is being written. You're probably thinking, "Why is he talking about people who only *think* they're overweight? They have nothing to do with me! I'm part of the group that *is* actually overweight!

"And why is he saying that even if I am part of the overweight group, if I do everything right—if I listen to my Body Signals and eat well—I still might not lose weight! It's an outrage!"

Let me see if I can calm your indignation with a dose of the truth.

People, large or small, weigh what they weigh for many reasons. You've learned some of these reasons in previous chapters, but now you're going to learn the *big* one! The *crucial* one! The *unspoken* one— the one that nobody wants to talk about.

You already know that some people are larger than need be because they don't listen to their Body Signals. And you already know that some people are larger than need be because they eat foods that their particular metabolism may not be able to handle well (see chapter 11). But you may not know that *big, crucial, unspoken,* reason.

Many people are large because they're at their healthiest weight— the weight at which they are genetically and biochemically programmed to function optimally.

The Hard Truth

I'll lay odds that you're really stewing over this one. "Oh, n-o-o-o," you're thinking. "He's not going to try to tell me that I'm *not* too fat, is he? Pul-e-e-e-se! Is he going to try to convince me that I only *think* I'm too fat? Or that I weigh this much because I'm supposed to! Really! He's not going to try to tell me that I didn't make myself this way and therefore I can't fix it! Come on! Give me a break!"

And that's not all. Compounding your irritation and distress, you also suspect that I'm now contradicting my earlier guarantee. Didn't I promise that if you gained control of your Body Signals and your intake of fat-promoting food, you'd solve your weight problem?

The Contradiction Explained

Yes. You're right. I did.

But there is no contradiction.

Listen carefully: My claim, all along, has been that by responding to your Body Signals and controlling your intake of fat-promoting food, you will lose *excess* weight!

From either point of view—genetic/biochemical or just plain health—you may not have any excess weight to lose! Put quite simply: You actually may be heavy because you are supposed to be heavy. It may not be your behaviors (or absence of certain behaviors) that have brought you to this weight. And if that's the case, then changing your behaviors might not make you smaller. Changing to an Instinctive Eater may make you smaller, but only by a small amount.

Has it ever occurred to you that you might be at or near your healthiest physiological weight despite the fact that it doesn't conform to your aesthetic ideal—or to those unscientific height/weight charts? I'm sure it has.

Nonetheless, seeing it now in print must raise some very serious questions in your mind—serious enough for me to address them immediately.

1. If this is what I'm supposed to weigh—why?
2. How can you claim that I'm healthy at this weight when everyone says fat is dangerous?
3. If I'm not destined to lose weight, why should I bother exercising?
4. If I'm going to stay at this weight, why should I bother responding to my Body Signals?
5. How do I find out what I'm supposed to weigh—how do I know if I'm too fat?

Body-Signal Review

Before those questions are answered, let's take two hypothetical situations: (1) You respond to your Body Signals, but because you're already at your setpoint, you lose no weight, or (2) having responded to your Body Signals, you've lost all the weight you're going to lose.

Now let's review some of the principles you learned on your way to becoming an Instinctive Eater.

Entitlement. Once you understand that you are *entitled,* you can have all the benefits normally attributed to thinness at your current weight. That means that you accept yourself as valuable and worthy exactly as you are—right now! Neither you nor your body needs to be "fixed."

Acceptance. By accepting yourself, you achieve the freedom to act. Acceptance allows you to choose how to run your life. It permits, if not demands, that you define your appearance today as your current standard of beauty. And once you've chosen this standard as your truth, no one can either vote on you or disparage you.

Commitment to self-nurturance. You are free to define the operating framework of your life as the pursuit of answers to these two questions: "What's best for *me?*" and "What nurtures *me?*" Your commitment to self-nurturance requires a commitment to caring for your body and attending to its health.

This Body-Signal review is most important for those of you who are at your ideal genetic/biochemical weight but *feel* as if you're too fat. You especially need to remember why it's crucial to respond to your Body Signals—whether you lose weight or not. Listen well.

Ignoring your Body Signals may or may not have made you fatter, but if you continue to ignore them, there is every chance in the world that you will erode your health!

Now let's tackle your questions.

Question 1: If This Is What I'm Supposed to Weigh—Why?

Before this can be answered, first you need to understand what fat is and how it works.

You and your fat. Fat, or adipose tissue, can be considered a distinct organ of the body. It is *not* a punishment for bad habits. To the contrary, fat has important functions and strong protective mechanisms. Its major function is energy storage.

Using rats as their models to learn about fat, researchers have conducted scores of studies in which the strength of our fat-defense mechanisms have been demonstrated. For instance, if you starve a rat, the size of each fat cell will be reduced, but not the number of fat cells. Researchers have found that when starvation is continued in genetically fat rats, muscle and brain are sacrificed before fat. The body fiercely holds on to its fat. (But then, you didn't need a rat study to tell you that, did you?)

Fat and the brain. Why is it that the body fights to keep its fat? Research studies indicate that an important function of the brain is to make sure that we neither gain nor lose too much weight. To this end, the brain aids in ensuring that we stay at the weight for which we're genetically programmed.

The research demonstrating this concept is fascinating. The brain has a pea-sized control center called the hypothalamus. Initial studies showed that when a portion of the hypothalamus—the ventromedial nucleus (VMH)—was damaged during the experiment, the subjects of the experiment overate and became obese. The logical conclusion of the research was that the VMH controlled satiety and therefore weight.

It just so happens that the "logical conclusion" was wrong. Experimentally induced damage to another region, the lateral hypothalamus (LH), caused the opposite effects—the subjects stopped eating, starved themselves, and lost weight. The logical conclusion of *this* research proved that the LH controls appetite and therefore weight.

Again, it just so happens that the "logical conclusion" was wrong.

Subsequent studies involving the VMH and LH proved that control of eating and fat was much more complex. It appears that the VMH and the LH don't control satiety and appetite, but rather body weight. Let me explain.

A healthy rat is supposed to weigh a certain amount. If its VMH is damaged, it will overeat until it achieves a higher weight. In other words, it would seem that the VMH is the rat's weight-control thermostat. Damage it and the "setting" will lock in at a higher weight. It will have a higher setpoint.

Now look what happens to a fat rat. If you damage its VMH, it will just *stay* fat. It won't overeat and get fatter—it will eat just enough to maintain the weight of this higher level. As a matter of fact, if the rat is too fat before you damage the VMH, it actually will undereat and lose some weight! Why? Because it wants to get to the new setpoint determined by the now-damaged VMH.

LH-damaged animals show the same effect in the opposite direction. Animals that have not been prestarved will undereat and lose weight. But if an LH-damaged animal has been prestarved, it will either eat vigorously or show no change. In other words, an already-thin rat won't lose weight when the LH is damaged.

What does this information suggest?

Since a prefattened VMH-damaged rat doesn't gain weight, and a prestarved LH-damaged rat doesn't lose weight, it just may be that the hypothalamus does *not* control appetite and satiety. *It just may be that the job of the hypothalamus is to defend body weight—as it is!*

What this means to you. The personal implication of these experiments is this: *Eating is determined by body weight—body weight isn't determined by eating.*

Brain damage seems to have little effect on hunger or satiety. It simply alters the weight that the animal will defend. These studies are important. They also show that body weight can change dramatically when eating remains unchanged! Think about it. All your life, you've been told that your weight is a result of how much you eat. Let's look at how these studies contradict that age-old notion.

Since a VMH-damaged animal gains weight, and an LH-damaged animal loses weight, you'd assume the VMH-damaged animal gains *all* its weight by overeating. Likewise, you'd assume that the LH-damaged animal loses *all* its weight by undereating. Neither is the case.

If the VMH-damaged animal is prevented from overeating, it still gains weight much faster than normal animals—and almost all the weight gained is fat.

If the LH-damaged animal is force-fed, it still loses weight.

What does this imply for you? That people can become fat not because they are gluttons but because their hypothalamus is "set" to maintain a certain weight with about the same food intake as a that of smaller person.

Let me complete the picture. These studies also imply that some people have a weight that is "set" so low, it's possible for them to eat large amounts without gaining.

Fat and energy. But your hypothalamus is not the whole story.

Dieters believe that weight control is governed by the equation: Calories (or energy) in equals calories out:

$$E \; In \; = \; E \; Out$$

They believe that if you decrease the energy you put in your body, or increase the energy your body expends, you'll lose the weight.

As you've discovered for yourself, this equation is more complicated than it appears. Here's the true equation:

$$E \; In \; = \; E \; Out \; (exercise) \; + \; E \; Out \; (metabolism)$$

The only form of *E In*, of course, is food. *E Out*—energy expenditure—occurs in *two* ways. *E Out* is voluntary (exercise) and involuntary (referred to as metabolic rate). The latter accounts for about 80 percent of *E Out*.

Metabolic rate, then, is the primary factor determining weight. If your involuntary energy expenditure—your metabolism—is slow, you can get fat *without overeating or underexercising.*

These three factors—eating, exercise, metabolic rate—interact in complex ways.

A quick look at thermogenesis. For instance, look at the difference between a starving person and a fed person. Feed a starving person, and she will use virtually all of the food energy to maintain voluntary and involuntary body functions—to keep the heart pumping, the lungs breathing, the body temperature regulated, and so forth. You could say that a starving person uses food (energy) with almost 100 percent efficiency.

A fed person, on the other hand, will "waste" a certain portion of the food energy by converting it into heat—or "burning it off." This process is called diet-induced thermogenesis, and it refers to the heat burned off by the body as it processes the food we've eaten.

To sum up so far, when you eat, the food will be used as energy (for either voluntary or metabolic activities), stored (including storage as fat), or wasted (burned off).

Thermogenesis and your weight. Diet-induced thermogenesis defends against large increases in body weight. The more calories burned, the less stored as fat. Young people, particularly teenagers, have very efficient thermogenic mechanisms that prevent weight gain. Unfortunately, since this wonderful efficiency can decline with age, fatness can increase with age.

But now let's take a look at how thermogenesis works.

- In one experiment, pigs were fed a protein-deficient diet and had to eat five times more food to get adequate protein. Still, they metabolically burned off the excess calories and gained no more weight than pigs on a normal diet. This particular experiment demonstrates not only the power of the thermogenic mechanism but also the body's defense of setpoint.
- In another study, rats genetically bred to be fat readily converted food into fat but were very poor at producing heat—or burning off the food they ate.
- In still another study, a comparison of fat and thin people was conducted. After a test meal, the fat people had a smaller increase in involuntary energy expenditure. Even after weight loss, the fatter people maintained a lower thermogenic response, which means they were storing more energy as fat.

When you think about it, you'll also begin to understand why it's so difficult for a heavy person who has lost weight to maintain the

---

BROWN FAT, MUSCLES, AND THERMOGENESIS

Brown fat, a specialized form of adipose tissue, is a powerful thermogenic tissue. Although a major controversy surrounds the role of brown fat in weight, a decline in human brown fat does occur around age 30 (a time when many people notice a weight gain). Another postulated thermogenic site is skeletal muscle, which would mean that our muscles are involved in both voluntary and involuntary energy expenditure.

weight loss. Not only is setpoint working against her, but the thermogenic response is as well.

What do these studies suggest?

It just could be that the conversion of food to heat plays a major role in determining whether a person will be fat or thin.

Let's return now to our weight-control equation:

$$E\ In\ =\ E\ Out\ (voluntary)\ +\ E\ Out\ (involuntary)$$

Here's what we've learned.

1. We can control $E\ In$ (food intake).
2. We can control, to a certain extent, $E\ Out$ (voluntary— exercise and activity).
3. We can't control $E\ Out$ (involuntary—metabolic rate). We can't control the percentage of our food that thermogenesis will burn off and the percentage that will be stored.

Since thermogenesis plays a major role in number 3, and since we can't control thermogenesis, we have one more reason that we can't necessarily weigh what we want to weigh.

You and weight. Why else do you weigh what you weigh? There are many different factors. Consider these findings.

Heredity. Perhaps the major factor behind your weight is heredity. Researchers have found that offspring of two fat parents have an 80 percent chance of being fat; with one fat parent, they have a 50 percent chance; if neither parent is fat, they have a 10 percent chance. Studies of twins (particularly twins separated at birth) have verified the heredity factor.

Nutritional stress. During pregnancy, nutritional stress can also play a role in determining your weight. Research shows that mothers who experienced either rapid weight gain or starvation in early pregnancy were more likely to have fat children.

Bottle-feeding. Infant feeding, too, may influence later weight. Bottle-fed babies weigh more than breast-fed babies. A breast-fed infant will respond to his or her Body Signals and stop sucking when satisfied. Bottle-fed babies are frequently encouraged to finish the whole bottle, which fosters overeating. Of course, infants can do little to compensate for overfeeding.

You also may be interested in knowing that cow's milk has different proteins than human milk and that infant formulas are often sweetened. These two factors could override a baby's Satisfaction Signal, causing overfeeding. Without knowing it, you may be nurturing a little Overeater!

Gender. Fatness is also affected by gender. The average male body is 20 percent fat; the average female body is 30 percent fat. Since a woman's metabolism is different from a man's, a woman is twice as likely to be fat. A woman who is heavy must understand that it's not her fault! Further, she would certainly be justified in telling her skinny husband to "knock it off" when he begins with that nonsense, "It's only a matter of willpower." (Interestingly, women still live substantially longer than men. When he starts on you, tell him that!)

Age. Here's another factor. The older you get, the fatter you get. However, you might find this additional piece of information puzzling: In the last 30 years, people have gotten fatter, food intake has *decreased,* and life expectancy has increased.

Nonfactors for fat. Setpoint. Thermogenesis. Heredity. Nutritional stress. Gender. Bottle-feeding. Age. With all of these factors, you must be wondering where numero uno comes in, right? What about good old overeating? Everyone knows that overeating is a factor in fatness, right?

Well, there's little evidence to support this notion. In fact, much of the available data show that fat people eat less than thin people! (It's kind of mind-boggling, isn't it?)

Still, it makes sense if they're thermogenically "burning off" less. Fatter people would naturally eat less because they use more of what they eat than their thinner counterparts. For example, a study of middle-aged men in Holland showed that the fattest men ate 20 to 25 percent less than the thinnest!

The belief that overeating is responsible for why you weigh what you weigh extracts a terrible toll on larger people. You weigh what you weigh because of a variety of factors that are completely out of your control. Still, no one acknowledges these unspoken factors. Instead, nonfactors such as overeating and underexercising are usually blamed. As a result, in an attempt to master factors that are outside the realm of control, the larger person jeers at her body, tries to torture it into submission, and endures enormous amounts of frustration and shame.

A self-fulfilling prophecy. Reading the height/weight charts can make fatter people even more discouraged by their repeatedly failed efforts to reach "normality." Feeling condemned to a life of "unhealthy fat," they can, and often do, develop defeatist attitudes. They may end up ignoring their Body Signals, abandoning nutritional good sense, eating a lot of fat and sugar, and neglecting exercise. As a result, it's quite possible that the "heavy" person of yesterday becomes the "heavier" person today.

Why did this happen?

Because no one told them they were essentially normal and healthy the way they were!

Question 2: How Can You Claim That I'm Healthy at This Weight When Everyone Says Fat Is Dangerous?

Let's take a look at the facts behind what "everyone says." There's some impressive evidence that everyone may be wrong.

Height/weight mythology. The weight-for-age and weight-for-height charts say nothing about whether fat is a health hazard. What they do say is that heavier people who take out life insurance are poorer risks.

The absurdity of using these charts as a health indicator was recently made evident in the United States. Do you remember this one? One day the charts were revised, and overnight millions of "endangered," "unhealthy" Americans became risk-free and healthy!

There are, in fact, many serious pitfalls in using these charts to assess health. This one is major: Just as there is no way to define normal or ideal weight, *there is no adequate definition of overweight.*

The now-famous Build and Blood Pressure Study reflected some important information about fat and health—or, to be more accurate, about fat and health *statistics.*

To get a better picture of that "important information," just for the fun of it, stop for a moment and take this multiple-choice quiz. All you have to do is circle the correct answer.

1. Blood pressure
   (*a*) Tall people are more likely to have high blood pressure.
   (*b*) Short people are more likely to have high blood pressure.
2. Fat
   (*a*) Ten percent of Americans are too fat.
   (*b*) Thirty-five percent of Americans are too fat.

If you circled (*a*) for questions 1 and 2, you are right. If you circled (*b*) for questions 1 and 2, you are also right.

Depending on how the statistics were viewed, the Build and Blood Pressure study arrived at both of these absurd conclusions for the first question. This particular study also showed that 10 percent of Americans are too fat, while the Metropolitan Life Insurance tables, using the same criteria, came to the conclusion that 35 percent of Americans were too fat.

If these conclusions confuse you, here's why: *A statistical analysis as applied to weight and health is basically irrelevant. There is no such thing as "normal" weight. Each individual has his or her own normal weight!*

The absurdity is further compounded. Can you imagine anyone using tables based on insurance policies held by upper middle-class Anglo-Saxon males living in Northeastern United States cities who were substantially lighter than the general population to determine the effect of fat on your health or mine?

Yes, it *is* ridiculous! You must bear in mind that the experts claim it's not weight per se that's the health culprit, but fat. After all, no one worries about the health of those 260-pound football behemoths. Therefore, if your fat content can't be measured, how can anyone tell you that you have too much unhealthy fat?

Unless you are willing to put your body in a giant blender and extract the fat with special solvents, you may never know what the exact percentage is. None of the measures for body fat percentage is really accurate.

Again—if we don't know what percentage of your weight is fat, how can we say your fat is unhealthy? (For the sake of accuracy, please note: If indirect measurements indicate that half of a person's body composition is fat, greater health risks are predicted for this select group.)

If you are healthy at your normal weight, then what is the real truth about the risks of fat to your health?

Fat and health. Yes, it's true that fatter people are more likely to have diabetes, high blood pressure, hyperlipidemia (elevated cholesterol and/or triglyceride levels), and heart disease.

We physicians preach that all overweight people should lose weight. Yet there is no good evidence that weight loss is beneficial for the vast majority of overweight people without these diseases. Because there is no good evidence, physicians should not only be reluctant to recommend weight loss for someone who is "overweight," we also should be very careful when we recommend weight loss for our patients who do have these conditions.

Let me explain.

It is likely that fatness does *not* cause diabetes and high blood pressure, but that diabetes and high blood pressure cause fatness. It's also likely that weight gain, not fatness, may precipitate these conditions.

While weight gain does appear to encourage diabetes and high blood pressure, it has not been clearly shown to bring about elevated cholesterol or triglyceride levels. However, weight gain is often associated with high fat intake, which *can* exacerbate hyperlipidemia.

In fact, most of the evidence that's in shows that body weight has little effect on health or life expectancy!

The Framingham Study, a long-term study of the relationship between body weight and heart disease in over 5,000 people from the town of Framingham, Massachusetts, showed the highest mortality for the thinnest men! The second highest mortality was for the very fattest. Between these two extremes, body weight had little effect on mortality.

Fat and the heart. Yes, people with diabetes, high blood pressure, and hyperlipidemia are more prone to heart attack. But a fat person with none of these conditions is no more likely to have a heart attack than a thin person!

The Framingham data showed a statistically significant relationship between weight and heart disease. What few people understand is that "statistically significant" means there's a difference between the risk of heavier people and lighter people. It doesn't say what that difference is. In this case, it turned out to be $\frac{1}{100}$ of 1 percent!

Statistically significant—yes. Medically significant—no!

Contrary to conventional thinking, numerous studies have shown that fat is *not* associated with cardiovascular mortality (except in the highest percentiles of weight). These studies included the classic Seven Countries Study, studies from southern Europe, studies from Finland, studies on 866 American soldiers, and a study of more than 12,000 white, middle-aged American men. If fat is really the lethal disease the doomsayers claim it is, how do we explain the fact that in the United States, cardiovascular mortality is decreasing as fatness is increasing?

What amazes me is how—in the absence of scientific support— fat bigotry continues to pervade our culture.

Fat and high blood pressure. Yes, again, fat is associated with high blood pressure. But again, the connection is not as simple as you've been led to believe. Consider these two findings.

- Highly developed societies that have a large population of fat people have high prevalence rates of hypertension, while underdeveloped societies with few fat people show very low rates.
- Rapid weight gain in young adults *is* a serious risk factor for developing high blood pressure.

These findings argue for the fact that fat causes high blood pressure. Other findings argue that fat does *not* cause high blood pressure. Here's what they show.

- Most fat people have normal blood pressures.
- Weight loss doesn't lower blood pressure for many people.
- People with high blood pressures are more prone to weight gain. (The reasons are unclear.)

While we can say that if you're fat, you're more likely to have high blood pressure, we can by no means conclude that you have high blood pressure because you're fat.

There are several possible reasons that fat people are more likely to have high blood pressures. The fact that people with high blood pressures are more prone to weight gain suggests one of these reasons— that fat and high blood pressure are symptoms of an as-yet-undiscovered common factor. In other words, the part of your genetic makeup that dictates you will be fat may also dictate that you'll have high blood pressure. (Tricky, isn't it?)

Other possible reasons?

- High blood pressure may be fostered by the composition of the diet that fat people eat (see chapter 11).
- Fat people are more likely to diet, and the diet/binge cycle can cause high blood pressure.
- In their efforts to change their shapes, many fat people ignore their Body Signals. As you've already learned, putting food into a body that isn't calling for fuel stimulates the sympathetic nervous system, which can cause high blood pressure.

Fat and diabetes. Yes, again, it's true: Fatness makes diabetes worse. And losing weight makes it better. Let me explain why.

Two of insulin's major functions are to transport excess blood sugar (glucose) out of the bloodstream into the cells and to store food as fat. In diabetics, the former is impaired and the latter isn't.

The result is a vicious cycle. To lower blood sugar, the pancreas secretes more insulin. But this is where the process boomerangs. Greater insulin secretion also promotes more fat storage, but higher amounts of body fat cause insulin resistance. (Insulin resistance means the cells resist the effect of insulin to transport the sugar out of the bloodstream.)

What's the end result? The body secretes more insulin, and as the insulin drives the blood sugar down, it drives the body fat up.

It's true that weight loss decreases insulin resistance. As a result, you would think (as your doctor does) that weight loss would be a good treatment for diabetes. But diabetics have a different metabolism from nondiabetics. For them, losing weight is much more difficult.

A doctor who puts a diabetic on a weight-loss diet is probably causing more harm than good. For one reason (which is the same for diabetics as it is for nondiabetics), diets are more likely to make you fatter than thinner.

For another reason, dieting, of course, is very stressful. It can cause the release of the stress hormone, adrenaline, which actually opposes the action of insulin. The diabetic can wind up defeating her own purposes.

Weight loss through dieting therefore is not a practical alternative for diabetics. There is some good news, however. Many diabetics can experience dramatic improvement without having to diet away an ounce. It turns out that exercise provides a powerful bonus—it decreases insulin resistance, therefore blood sugar is reduced.

I might also add at this point that exercise appears to help high blood pressure and high cholesterol. A study in Sweden found that hypertensive women who were placed on an exercise program dropped their blood pressures—even though weight wasn't lost. Exercise has also been shown to increase HDL cholesterol—the "good" cholesterol that protects you from heart disease.

And those aren't the only benefits of exercise.

HOW TO TALK TO YOUR DOCTOR ABOUT HIGH BLOOD PRESSURE AND DIABETES

If you're overweight and have high blood pressure and/or diabetes, your physician will undoubtedly tell you to lose weight. In response, tell your doctor that the most recent research shows that if you do attempt to lose weight, you're more likely to aggravate the problem.

What your doctor probably has in mind is a diet or some type of calorie restriction. By now, you know that following through on this recommendation usually produces results that are precisely the opposite of what you hoped for.

Tell your doctor that your high blood pressure may be a result of your genetics, not your weight. If the doctor is up on the literature on hypertension, she will know that obesity is actually a protective factor. In other words, fat people with high blood pressures are not as likely to suffer the same consequences as thinner people with high blood pressures.

Tell your doctor that if the condition isn't genetic, it may be a result of the content of your diet, your past efforts at dieting (with the subsequent bingeing and overeating), or because you never learned to respond to your Body Signals.

Tell her that before you concentrate on your weight, you'd like to focus your attention on changing your eating habits and that you want her support in this endeavor. While you're at it, explain the importance of listening to your Body Signals—and why you think that's the soundest initial approach to treating your high blood pressure and diabetes.

Most books you read tell you not to treat yourself without a doctor's supervision. I'm saying something slightly different. I'm saying don't treat yourself without a doctor's collaboration.

Question 3: If I'm Not Destined to Lose Weight, Why Should I Bother Exercising?

You can't dismiss an understanding of the results of exercise, regardless of the role it plays in paring off pounds.

Exercise and weight. "I know that's not the only benefit of exercise," you're probably thinking, "but exercise is essential if I want to lose weight."

Sorry, it's just not so. Exercise has a lot of health benefits, but it turns out that significant weight loss is really not one of them.

Let me explain why exercise has very little impact on weight.

As you've already learned, *E In* and *E Out* are influenced by each other. Reduce your activity, and you'll wind up eating less; increase it, and you'll eat more. Basically, it balances out. You might feel like you're eating less on the days you go to your aerobics class, but studies show that after a certain point, as your activity levels increase, so does your food consumption.

Now you're probably thinking, "This contradicts everything I've ever learned about exercise and weight. Are you trying to convince me that exercise doesn't burn off calories? I know you must be wrong, because just this week I saw a chart in a magazine and another one above the stationary bicycle in my health club—both showed how many extra calories my exercise was burning off."

These charts may be valid except that they assume that when you're not exercising, you're comatose! The truth is, even when you're not exercising, you're expending a great deal of energy merely to stay alive.

The notion that you can dramatically increase your energy expenditure and burn off more calories is wrong. You already use so much energy for your metabolic processes and your ordinary daily activities that when you add exercise, it hardly makes a dent. For example, if you climbed the highest mountain in Britain, you would increase your energy expenditure by about 22 percent.

"Well, that's not so awful," you're probably thinking. True, but it still isn't great. Depending on how active you are, if you climb that mountain you'll increase your daily energy expenditure by less than 100 to several hundred kilocalories (kcal). Since you need to expend 4,000 kcal to burn off a pound of fat, you'd have to climb that mountain every day for weeks just to burn off a pound—and that assumes that you wouldn't allow yourself extra rest after your climb.

There are some other reasons why exercise does not take off the pounds.

- When you rest after exercise, you're possibly using lower energy levels than you would if you hadn't exercised.
- Sometimes exercise can trigger increased food intake.
- The more we exercise, the more we train our muscles to be efficient. (With efficient muscles, less effort is required to produce the same result, so less energy is burned off.)
- It appears that the better trained we are through exercise, the more efficient our diet-induced thermogenesis mechanism becomes. As a result, we burn off fewer calories.

I don't want to discourage you from exercising. But I do want to discourage you from overexercising because you're motivated by misinformation.

Yes, exercise can have positive impact on weight, which probably occurs in two ways, directly and indirectly.

The direct impact was shown in studies that demonstrated an increase in metabolic rate. Some of these studies showed that this effect could last for up to 15 hours after exercise. Regular aerobic exercise (perhaps 30 to 40 minutes four times a week) can, therefore, lower setpoint, not by burning off calories but by increasing metabolic rate. However, this reduction appears to be somewhat insubstantial. Researchers found that in the fattest people, exercise appeared to lower stable weight by a maximum of 12 pounds—which appears to be the most weight you can lose directly through exercise.

Indirect effects of exercise and body signals. My co-author, Gail, who takes exercise seriously, also took indignant exception to this information.

"I insisted Steve tell me how he could claim that exercise doesn't cause weight loss when there are so many women at my gym who tell me they've lost 20, 40, 60 pounds through regular workouts. How is it that my 'real life' experience could so completely contradict the scientific evidence?"

There was only one explanation I could give her—and you. I'm not saying that exercise has no effect on weight, I'm simply saying that the effect is rather insignificant—*unless you consider the possible indirect effects!*

Think about what happens to people who are totally committed to their exercise programs. Is it likely that they will:

- Exercise in a vacuum—that the exercise will be an isolated activity having no effect on the other parts of their lives?
- Continue to binge and overeat?
- Go on eating junk food?
- Keep feeling out of control?

- Continue to let the Internal Saboteur run their lives?
- Go on undervaluing themselves and neglecting self-nurturance?
- Continue to ignore their Body Signals?

No—not bloody likely.

Exercise and the Internal Saboteur. When you carry out your commitment to exercise, you're nurturing your body. When you nurture your body, you're nurturing yourself. Exercise is crucial because it's a constant reminder that you and your body are one; that when you care for your body, you're caring for *you!*

The Internal Saboteur will always attempt to undermine your efforts to care for yourself. It conducts guerrilla warfare, sending insidious messages and images intent on crippling your resolve.

But when you exercise, the Internal Saboteur is forced into face-to-face, down-and-dirty combat with you. For instance, you decide to jog 3 miles and step out smartly. But with every step, it's asking you, "Why bother?" At this point, it's now you versus it. When you complete your 3 miles and you know you've won, you feel terrific. And that triumph isn't isolated. Exercise victories over the Internal Saboteur "ripple" into other aspects of your life.

This dynamic is critical. Becoming a person who responds to her Body Signals is a major lifestyle change. The impulse to return to compulsive eating will linger for some time—the Internal Saboteur will repeatedly try to defeat your efforts. But every time you exercise and beat it at its game, your power over its messages is reinforced. Ultimately, its attempts to undermine your new, healthy eating habits will have less impact and less potency.

MAJOR BENEFITS OF EXERCISE

- Lowers pulse rate and increases the amount of blood pumped to the body
- Modifies Type-A behavior
- Increases cholesterol solubility, and as a result, lowers the risk of gallstones
- Decreases the risks of osteoporosis
- Increases T-cell (immune cell) production
- Stabilizes moods/depression
- Reduces occurrence of viral illnesses as such as colds and flu
- Possibly affects longevity

Question 4: If I'm Going to Stay at This Weight, Why Should I Bother Responding to my Body Signals?

Maintaining a stable weight has advantages not readily apparent to the casual observer.

Overweight versus weight gain. As you've learned, except in the very thinnest and very fattest groups, weight is not a health risk per se. Yet heavier people do indeed have a higher incidence of high blood pressure, diabetes, and high cholesterol.

Why?

Since it's not their weight, and since it's not because they eat too much, we have to look for other culprits.

Two come to mind: overeating and weight fluctuations. (Let me make a note here: In this context, overeating doesn't mean eating too much. It means eating when your body isn't signaling you to eat.)

Consider these findings.

Take two groups of people: One group has been obese since childhood; the other became obese as adults. The former group has stable obesity; the latter group demonstrates weight gain, very likely from overeating. When you compare the two groups, you'll find an increased incidence of cardiovascular disease in the group that overate and gained weight as adults.

Now take two different groups: overweight adults who were overweight children, and overweight adults who were underweight children. The former group—again with stable obesity—has the same incidence of high blood pressure as average-weight adults. The group that moved from underweight to overweight has a higher incidence of high blood pressure.

These facts seem to indict overeating and weight gain as a cause of high blood pressure.

Now let's take a look at weight loss.

You know that weight loss is often associated with a reduction in high blood pressure. What has not been determined, however, is whether the subsequent decline in blood pressure is a result of the weight loss or is a result of the cessation of overeating.

Overweight versus overeating. A good case can be made for the cessation of overeating as the answer.

You may recall that studies in humans show that overeating releases the stress hormone noradrenalin, which raises pulse rate, blood pressure, and metabolic rate.

The increased metabolic rate burns off the extra calories from the binge. For this reason, Instinctive Eaters who only pig out on rare occasions do not gain weight.

With repeated episodes of overeating, however, the effect of noradrenalin on metabolic rate is extinguished. But its effect on pulse and blood pressure persists.

This may mean that if you're fat because you're at setpoint, then you're healthy. But if you're fat because you overeat, then you may be at risk.

Support for this idea is found in studies showing that insulin resistance and diabetes have a closer correlation to overeating than to overweight. Experimental evidence indicates that it is weight fluctuations that predispose us to impaired glucose tolerance. Similarly, increasing serum lipids (cholesterol, triglycerides, and the like) had a closer correlation to increased caloric intake than to weight.

A Nurses' Health Study followed 115,886 healthy women aged 30 to 55, and the results, published in the *New England Journal of Medicine,* appeared to support the idea that being fatter increased a woman's risk of heart attack. Women who were 30 percent (or more) overweight

BODY SIGNALS AND HEALTH

People who listen to their Body Signals get hungry several times a day (not just the traditional three!). Take a look at these findings.

- In a study of 379 men ages 60 to 64, those who ate three meals a day—as compared to those who ate five or more smaller meals—showed excessive weight gain, increased cholesterol levels, and decreased glucose tolerance.
- More frequent feedings have been shown to cause increased resistance to obesity, atherosclerosis, and diabetes. When they eat more frequently, patients with these conditions respond better to their specific therapies.
- Studies of rats and chickens showed that large meals ingested by these animals once or twice a day elevated their serum cholesterol levels and increased their incidence and severity of atherosclerosis.
- People who changed from the customary three meals a day to six smaller feedings showed a drop in cholesterol.
- Animals that take all their food in one meal are more likely to get fat than those that eat the same amount in a series of snacks.

tripled their risk. For 70 percent of the women with heart disease, over-weight played a role. The questions still remain: Was it the weight itself that caused the heart disease? Or was it overeating and weight gain that promoted these frightening statistics?

One final statistic might provide a good clue. That same study showed that women who gained more than 20 pounds after age 18 doubled their risk of heart disease.

Fortunately, the study also showed that taking action against this battle of the bulge was beneficial. However, if you are in this cate-gory, taking action does *not* mean dieting (see "Overweight versus Weight Fluctuations" below). It does mean listening to your Body Signals.

The Body-Signal necessity. After looking at all this information, we can reasonably conclude:

- The body knows what it should weigh.
- The body has all the tools it needs to maintain this weight.
- If the body is not extremely thin or extremely fat and does maintain this weight, it will be healthy—no matter what that weight is.
- If we listen to what the body tells us—our Body Signals—then we will enjoy good health because we will be at our best weight.
- What you weigh doesn't matter as long as your weight stays stable.

OVERWEIGHT VERSUS
WEIGHT FLUCTUATIONS

Here are some fascinating findings on how loss-and-gain cycles affect health.

- Animal studies inducing cycles of weight loss/weight gain re-sulted in hypertension, heart disease, and shortened life span.
- After the semistarvation siege of Leningrad in 1942, when food supplies were restored, the prevalence of hypertension quadrupled.
- In a medically supervised fast regimen in Los Angeles, a group of overweight veterans experienced a cycle of loss/regain, loss/regain. Eighty percent developed diabetes and 25 percent died—predominantly from heart disease. This death rate was 13 times higher than that of equally overweight nondieters who were fol-lowed in Denmark and Norway.

Question 5: How Do I Find Out What I'm Supposed to Weigh— How Do I Know If I'm Too Fat?

Listen to your Body Signals. Your body will take you to your "right" weight as though you were a passenger on the Concorde. Don't worry about whether you're too fat, because even if you are, if you listen to your Body Signals, you'll lose your excess weight. Don't concern yourself with weight, don't concern yourself with fat, don't concern yourself with scales, don't concern yourself with height/weight charts, don't concern yourself with calories—if you must concern yourself with something, just keep your focus on your eating and your Body Signals.

Chapter 11

Body-Signal Interference: Foods That Fatten

Dieters worry about the taboo of fattening foods. I've never yet met a dieter who knows what really makes a food fattening.

The connection between what goes on in real life and the scientific findings that confirm our everyday experiences is often obscure to those who have no laboratory background. Let me illustrate how science proves the value of my Body-Signal Program.

Real Life

A few years ago, a woman named Karen showed up at a Lighten Up seminar waxing ecstatic about the 100 pounds she had lost on a "diet." When she didn't receive the expected raves, Karen was extremely put out. But then something fascinating occurred. While being questioned about her "diet"—what she ate and didn't eat—Karen indignantly explained that she had given up all sugar and only ate nutritious foods.

"That was no *diet*," we all exclaimed, "that was Instinctive Eating!"

Susan, a seminar support team leader who refers to herself as a reformed "chocoholic," took the seminar in 1985 as a size 16. Since that weekend, she has gained control of her sugar intake, gone down to a size 8, and remained there.

As for me, the Italian bakery near my home sells not only mouth-watering pastries and delicious-looking chocolate goodies but also a splendid variety of Italian ices and ice creams. Occasionally, while walking past that bakery in the evening, I'd think my body was signaling a need for a piece of chocolate cake.

I was wrong.

Why did Karen and Susan lose so much weight simply by controlling sugar?

And how did I know I was receiving a false Body Signal?

Foods That Fatten

It's pretty unlikely that Susan and Karen would have lost any weight if they had continued to eat excessive amounts of sugar. And it is also pretty unlikely that people who receive false Body Signals (like mine) and don't recognize their falseness will reach their optimal weight.

During the first 30 years of my life, I ate hundreds and hundreds of pounds of sugar. Now when I find myself in situations like the one in front of the bakery, I don't know if I really want the chocolate cake or if the wires to my Hunger Signals have gotten crossed. I know that many times they are crossed, because when I eat "real" food, my craving for sugar disappears. This is how I've come to recognize the falseness of my sugar signal. It's not false all of the time—but it is false a lot of the time.

If my body is hungry, but I think it just wants a "sweet fix," then I have to conclude that all those years of eating sugar have created these crossed wires that interfere with my true Body Signals. I admit this is not science—it's only my opinion based on my personal and professional experience with patients and seminar participants.

No, it's not necessarily the calorie content in sugar that makes people fatter. I suspect that people who eat too much sugar grow fatter because sugar appears to have properties that distort our Body Signals and make us overeat. In fact, nutritional scientists are now asking questions like these:

• Are there indeed foods that can make you fat, independent of their caloric content?
• How do these foods manage to fatten you?
• If you avoid or cut down on these foods, will you promote weight loss?
• Even if your weight may not change, if you cut down on these foods, will your health improve?

At present, the answers to these questions are by no means conclusive. But there is a measure of circumstantial evidence that would indict, if not convict, the following dietary substances.

- Sugar
- Artificial sweeteners
- Dietary fat
- "Enriched" white flour
- Alcohol
- Fried foods

Science Life

You've seen what happened to Karen, Susan, and me in real life; now take a look at some interesting facts about these six substances.

Sugar. Interestingly, concomitant with a rise in sugar consumption, the incidence of obesity has risen tremendously in this century.

Artificial sweeteners. An American Cancer Society study of 78,694 women showed that those who used artificial sweeteners were significantly more likely to gain weight than nonusers—even though those who used the artificial sweeteners "ate chicken, fish, and vegetables significantly more often than did nonusers and consumed beef, butter, white bread, potatoes, ice cream, and chocolate significantly less often."

Dietary fat. At Cornell University, women eating a diet of varying fat content showed these responses:

- With 50 percent of the calories as fat, they ate 2,700 calories and put on ⅔ pounds in two weeks.
- With 33⅓ percent of the calories as fat, they ate 2,300 calories with no weight change.
- With 20 percent of the calories as fat, they ate 2,100 calories and lost almost a pound in two weeks.

It's interesting to note that the average American eats 40 percent of total food intake as fat.

"Enriched" white flour. Thirty-five overweight college students who believed they were participating in a nutrition experiment were actually taking part in a weight-control experiment in which they were allowed to make only one lifestyle change. They were to substitute whole-grain products for those made with refined, "enriched" white flour. At the end of three months, they each lost an average of 17½ pounds.

Alcohol. Here's a fast look at the calories that come with alcohol and other basic elements in foods.

Food Element	Calories per Ounce
Alcohol	240
Carbohydrate	130
Fat	310
Protein	140

Although fat contains more energy than alcohol, alcohol is absorbed more rapidly than other substances, and almost 100 percent of its energy is stored for utilization. In other words, calories from alcohol are not burned off!

Fried foods. Fried foods are the only item on our list that may make you fatter strictly because of calorie content.

The Body-Signal Sweetness Question

Forty volunteers at Yale University ate dinner, then fasted until they were given breakfast in a laboratory the next morning. The volunteers were divided into three groups, each to receive a single beverage: water, fructose (fruit sugar), or glucose syrup, which is sweeter than fructose.

Two hours and 15 minutes later, the volunteers were admitted to a buffet lunch, and after they ate, their calorie consumption was measured. The glucose group ate 450 more calories than the fructose group. (Just to illustrate a point, note that if all those calories were converted to body fat—which you've now learned doesn't happen—an extra 450 calories a day would translate into 50 pounds in a year!)

In my opinion, however, this was not the interesting part of the experiment. There was another dramatic finding.

Before lunch, the three groups were asked to rate their hunger on a scale of 0 to 4. Here's how they scored themselves: The water group, 4; the fructose group, 2; and the glucose group, 0.

That's right! The members of the glucose group—those who ate an extra 450 calories—were satiated before they sat down!

Yet they ate the most. Why?

A theory that has received widespread attention is that sweet substances either stimulate the appetite or block satiety—in other words, interfere with Body Signals.

If sweetness itself is the culprit, as this experiment suggests, then sucrose (table sugar) and artificial sweeteners might actually promote weight gain.

A Theoretical Example

Again, let's get personal. Just for a moment, let's suppose that at noon, you leave work and take off for lunch. During your meal, you drink an artificially sweetened soda, or maybe after your meal, you eat a sugared dessert.

It's now 2 hours later, and you're hungry again. Responding to your Body Signals, you eat something. Except in this case, maybe the Body Signal was "unnatural." I mean "unnatural" in that it might never have been "turned on" without the sweet consumption.

Do sweet substances move you to eat more? Do they make you fatter?

The Answer

It's not clear. Based on a comprehensive literature review, the Food and Drug Administration Sugars Task Force concluded that "sugars do *not* [italics added] have a unique role in the etiology of obesity."

Nonetheless, the case cannot be considered closed. It may be that sugar *does* play a less obvious role. Consider the possibility that:

- Sugar only appears to have no effect because it is one of several dietary factors that promote overeating.
- The form of sugar in the diet (*i.e.,* sugary drinks versus sugary foods) actually does play a role in determining its fattening effects.
- There may be individual differences in sugar (and fat) preferences and intakes.
- Athough obesity is understood to be primarily due to genetic make-up and may not actually be caused by eating sugar, the sugar may increase the *degree* of obesity.
- Individual responses are so variable that a uniform pattern doesn't emerge.

My Experience

I particularly favor the last explanation. In fact, my personal experience suggests it may indeed be valid.

When I turned 30, I moved to New York to start my internship. At that point, I immediately switched over to a classical junk food diet.

I'd buy a 64-ounce bottle of cola and work my way through it over a couple of days. I'd buy a box of cookies or cake and nibble throughout the day. Breakfast was a sugary cereal, milk, fried eggs, home fries, and white toast with butter. Lunch was blister-pack salami or bologna on white bread. Dinner was french fries and a hamburger on a white roll smothered in ketchup.

It wasn't long before I noticed I had developed a small potbelly. Yes, I was still thin, but I had acquired this 15-pound roll of fat that tumbled over my belt.

"Isn't this interesting!" I naively noted. "I arrive at age 30 and develop a potbelly."

Although my "pot" appeared suddenly, it never became any bigger. Then, two years later, as I finished my residency, I started to change my diet. In a very short time, without my even trying to get rid of it, my potbelly seemed to melt away.

Later on, I came to this conclusion: My body represents one end of a spectrum of possible responses to a diet loaded with sugar and/or fat and/or fried foods. This body will gain a finite amount of weight and stabilize at its new level.

Karen and Susan represent the other end of the spectrum. Their physiology is so sensitive to one or more of these substances that they will continue to gain as they continue to overeat these foods.

Sugar, Fat, and Setpoint

Support for the idea of individual susceptibility to sugar and/or fat comes from both animal and human studies. Rats have been studied using "cafeteria diets"—diets that sacrifice protein and complex carbohydrates for very high percentages of sugars (simple carbohydrates) and fats.

Cafeteria diets usually produce large increases in food intake and, eventually, substantial weight increases. If the animals have access to the cafeteria diet for only a short time, a return to their normal chow will produce voluntary undereating and rapid weight loss that brings them back to normal. The weight gained and lost is virtually all fat, which means that these diets are fat promoting.

If the rats stay on the cafeteria diet for a long time, many, but not all, appear to undergo a permanent change. A return to the old diet will result in increased food intake to defend the weight gain.

It could be said that a diet high in sugar and fat will produce an upward shift in setpoint.

The Fat Rats' Fate

The cafeteria diet increases the number of fat cells in the newly fat rats, and as you now know, new fat cells are permanent. The increase in fat cell number appears to parallel the upward shift in weight and setpoint.

Many species display the same pattern found in rats. While studies like this have not been conducted on humans, after prolonged exposure to "Western" diets, many groups around the world have displayed large increases in fatness. Again, in *susceptible* humans, the fat appears to be permanent.

The important point here is the variable response to these diets. Not everyone can anticipate a "fat fate." Some lab animals (and very likely humans, too) resist weight gain even when fed the richest of diets. Others become fat "junk food addicts."

When exposed to cafeteria diets, albino rats are an example of a strain that shows great variability in weight gain. Logic would suggest that humans, being much more genetically heterogeneous, would show an even greater variability.

Sweet Rats

Cafeteria diets include sugar and fat.

For now, let's just look at sugar and Body Signals. What can we conclude about that relationship? Let's peruse some intriguing research.

Experiments involving rats show that when they're given free access to both a sugar solution and standard laboratory chow, they'll consume approximately 60 percent of their calories as sugar, they'll overeat, and they'll become obese.

Another group of rats, given the choice of chow, water, and a sucrose solution, likewise consumed 50 to 60 percent of their calories as sugar (in other words, they ate only 40 to 50 percent as chow). By replacing 50 to 60 percent of chow with sucrose, they ultimately consumed 15 to 20 percent more calories.

Still another study showed that free access to sugar caused a significant increase in caloric intake. The rats ate 86 percent of their calories in the form of simple carbohydrates (sugars).

A rabbit study showed that just a few drops of a sweet-tasting glucose or fructose solution added to the diet stimulated a significant increase in subsequent chow intake.

If humans respond like rabbits, this could be especially important. In the United States, for example, the greatest increase in the consumption of sugar is in beverages—particularly soft drinks.

Humans are not laboratory animals. Still, these animal studies do show that adding sugar to the diet can increase calorie consumption, body weight, and body fat. Does this mean that we humans should be worried?

Probably so. If you look at the results of human studies, they're not so different from the animal studies. Let me explain.

Sweet Humans

A group of scientists was surprised to find that people eating the least amount of sugar on one diet lost more weight than people on another diet, despite the fact that the calories were equal. After all, it is known that diets of equal calories produce equal weight loss. In this instance, however, the dieters who lost less weight were on a diet with a higher sugar content.

The scientists felt that the low-sugar group lost more because their Hunger Signals were turned on less. Therefore, this group would be better able to stick to the diet than the high-sugar group.

Other studies also showed that dieters in the low-sugar groups had an easier time of it than dieters in the high-sugar groups. For example, subjects given low-fat, high-carbohydrate diets have reported that they were "discouraged" because they were always conscious of being hungry, while subjects given low-carbohydrate diets reported that they did not experience hunger. (This may ring true for you: If you've ever been on a low-carbohydrate diet, like the Scarsdale or the Atkins, you may have noticed that hunger wasn't a problem.)

In a similar example, a low-carbohydrate diet helped obese people control hunger better and achieve satiation. While fat, protein, and total calories were unrestricted, carbohydrates were restricted. Under these conditions, patients maintained prediet levels of fat and protein, but significantly reduced calories.

When the carbohydrate restriction was removed, the patients increased carbohydrate intake. But caloric intake increased beyond that attributable to the additional carbohydrate calories! What does this suggest? That simple carbohydrates have a stimulating effect on appetite and hunger.

If this is true, then it would be easier to reduce caloric intake by limiting sugar rather than fat, protein, complex carbohydrates, or calories in general.

Sugar and Body Signals

At one time, some scientists postulated that sugar ingestion triggered the following series of events.

1. Sight, smell, taste, and ingestion causes increased insulin levels (hyperinsulinemia).
2. Hyperinsulinemia drives down sugar in the bloodstream (hypoglycemia).
3. The brain registers the hypoglycemia and transmits appetite and Hunger Signals.
4. The body eats more food, particularly sugar.
5. Obesity results.

Subsequent scientific evidence doesn't support this simple pathway.

The Sugar Contradictions

Okay. Then how does sugar interfere with the Body Signals (if, in fact, it actually does)?

Many studies show that low blood sugar (hypoglycemia) is associated with hunger. But eating sweets in response to that hunger doesn't necessarily cause hypoglycemia. Insulin levels do increase with greater sugar consumption, but not usually enough to produce hypoglycemia.

What insulin has repeatedly been shown to do is produce hunger sensations and increased food intake and ultimately cause obesity. Chronic obesity is associated with higher insulin levels. When obese people see, smell, or eat food, they exhibit higher insulin levels than lean people. Additionally, they are frequently prone to insulin-induced hypoglycemia. Yet it must be noted that these differences are not true of *all* obese people and may reflect genetic predisposition rather than a response to eating too much sugar.

What we're left with is a measure of evidence that *in susceptible individuals,* overeating sugar can affect Body Signals and promote weight gain.

Artificial Sweeteners

Do artificial sweeteners interfere with Body Signals and make you fatter? The jury is out on this question.

Let's listen to the prosecution and the defense.

The prosecution points to epidemiological studies that have compared body weight, sugar intake, and artificial sweetener use. These studies have found that overweight generally goes with *lower* sugar intake but *greater* use of artificial sweeteners.

The defense, however, states that in older women on American diets, there is no real evidence that artificial sweeteners either increase or decrease food intake in a manner that affects obesity.

One study showed that eating sweets—whether artificial sweetener or sugar—seems to cause people to eat more. This study involved milkshakes that were sweetened with either sucrose or aspartame. These sweet milkshakes were compared with milkshakes in which the sweetness was suppressed by an added "sweet blocker."

After the subjects drank the milkshakes, they ate a test meal. Where the sweetness was *not* blocked, the subjects ate more. This would suggest that sweetness per se stimulates eating. An interesting additional finding was that the sweetness of the milkshakes also stimulated an increased consumption of other sweets.

On the other hand, again, when compared to sucrose, aspartame (which is sweeter than sucrose) has been shown to lower food intake. Normal-weight patients and obese patients were fed meals that contained sucrose. Later, aspartame was substituted for the sucrose. Both groups then dropped their daily caloric intake by 15 percent and maintained their new caloric levels.

While this study suggests that a diet containing aspartame will facilitate weight loss and maintenance compared to a diet containing sucrose, it does fail to answer an important question: If the subjects had stayed on the sucrose-containing meals, would they have eventually decreased their intake of calories as well?

In any event, it is reasonable to conclude that attempts to control weight by substituting artificial sweeteners is not likely to be successful. Long-term use has not been shown to help weight loss or prevent weight gain.

Sugar, Fat, and Thermogenesis

Up to this point, we've talked about the weight hazard of sugar and artificial sweeteners, meaning their effect on Body Signals. But the recent news indicts dietary fat as a greater weight hazard than sugar. Why? Because of the role that dietary fat plays in thermogenesis.

Did you know that it's easier to turn food fat into body fat than it is to turn carbohydrate into body fat?

Consider this: To store dietary fat as fat takes 3 percent of your thermogenic energy (the energy that it takes to digest the food); to store carbohydrate as carbohydrate (in a form called glycogen) takes 7 percent of your thermogenic energy; and to convert carbohydrate to body fat takes 23 percent of your energy.

As you can see, the body burns little thermogenic energy when it handles fat. Not only does it burn off much more energy changing carbohydrate to fat, but the body appears to resist doing it.

A group of healthy young people was fed 700 grams of carbohydrate—2,800 calories. Almost all of it was stored as glycogen. Look how much carbohydrate was eaten, and yet virtually none was stored as fat! It took a much greater level of carbohydrate intake to produce an increase in fat deposition.

The more carbohydrate you eat, the more you store and the more you burn.

This isn't true for fat. Subjects were fed the same breakfast, some with and some without an extra ten pats of margarine. The body didn't adjust to those ten extra pats by burning off the extra fat. Although the body will maintain carbohydrate and protein balance automatically, it doesn't work that way for fat.

Fat People and Fat Diets

Fatter people seem to prefer the taste of fat. They choose milkshakes with higher fat content than lean people. They don't eat more calories than lean people, but they do eat more of their calories as fat.

This apparent craving for fat may be linked to an enzyme called lipoprotein lipase (LPL), according to research at the University of Colorado Health Sciences Center. One of LPL's functions is to store fat in adipose (fat) cells. When a normal-weight person eats fat, LPL will decrease—the body tries to use the fat as energy before storing it.

When formerly obese women (whose LPL levels are already higher) eat fat, those already high levels rise higher still. In other words, by preferentially placing the fat calories into storage, formerly obese people react contrary to normal-weight people.

What's the upshot? Dietary fat appears to be particularly fat promoting in some larger people.

"Enriched" White Flour, Alcohol, and Fried Foods

Let me wind up my discussion about foods that fatten.

"Enriched" white flour. A second study (done at the University of Michigan) found results similar to those of the "enriched" flour study described earlier in which the students lost an average of 17½ pounds in three months by switching to whole grains. Why did whole grains produce these results? Two possible explanations come to mind.

One relates to the amount of insulin released when you eat a certain kind of food. "Enriched" white flour may trigger a response similar to sugar and likewise trigger hunger in a fashion similar to sugar.

The other proposed reason points out the effect of high fiber on appetite. Whole grains are high in fiber; "enriched" wheat has none. A high-fiber diet promotes satiety and a feeling of fullness more readily than a low-fiber diet. As a result, people eating a high-fiber diet may feel more satisfied with less food.

Alcohol. Because of the reasons mentioned earlier (alcohol is so easily absorbed in the stomach, and there's no thermogenic burning off of calories), I would argue that alcohol is the single most fattening substance.

Fried foods. Because frying a food greatly increases its caloric content, a diet of fried foods may promote weight gain.

However, the major menace of fried foods is not merely their high calorie counts. Fried foods appear to promote serious diseases.

As a matter of fact, to complete the picture, I need to shift my emphasis away from weight and provide you with some information concerning the possible health consequences of overeating sugar, fat, and fried foods.

The United States Senate's Select Committee

In July 1976, discussing the relationship of diet to disease, Mark Hegsted, M.D., of the Harvard School of Public Health, said the following:

> I wish to stress that there is a great deal of evidence, and it continues to accumulate, which strongly implicates, and in some instances proves, that the major causes of death and disability in the United States are related to our diet. I include coronary artery disease, which accounts for nearly half of the deaths in the United States, several of the most important forms of cancer, hypertension, diabetes, and obesity, as well as other chronic diseases.

The thrust of Dr. Hegsted's comments revolves around the composition of the standard American diet.

In the United States, Americans eat a diet of approximately 20 percent sugar and 40 percent fat. By far, most of the grains Americans eat are in the form of "enriched" refined wheat flour (white flour), which has been stripped of all vitamins, minerals, and fiber. In the processing plant, a minimum of three vitamins and one mineral (iron) is added back.

Depending on which statistics you analyze, the average American eats 70 to 120 pounds of refined sugar per year. To place that number in perspective, think about this:

- Six hundred years ago, the average consumption of sugar by all humans was zero! The refining processes hadn't yet been invented.
- In American Revolutionary War times, the average lifetime consumption of sugar was 500 pounds.
- Today, by the time we're in elementary school, we Americans have eaten more sugar than our Revolutionary War ancestors did in their entire lives!

Few people are fully aware of how much sugar they eat. After years of taking dietary histories, I have yet to encounter a single patient who realizes that she or he is eating almost ⅕ to ⅓ pound of sugar every day!

Sugar and Health

Sugar has been accused of aggravating just about every medical condition known, from arthritis to atherosclerosis, hemorrhoids to hypertension, constipation to cancer, dementia to diabetes, hiatal hernia to high cholesterol. But there is no hard proof that sugar plays a role in any of these conditions.

Yes, there is evidence that sugar can promote obesity, but there is no hard proof. Likewise, there is evidence that sugar can aggravate health problems—but again, we're without hard proof.

Sugar, Fat, and the Heart

The two most serious risk factors for heart disease (along with cigarette smoking) are a high cholesterol level and high blood pressure. There is evidence linking sugar consumption to these two conditions.

We know that dietary fat may aggravate a cholesterol problem. There is also evidence that sugar and fat combined may be more dangerous than fat alone. The evidence holds true for high blood pressure as well as high cholesterol.

Cafeteria diets given to rats were shown to stimulate sympathetic

THE EFFECT OF SUGAR ON BLOOD FATS

Table sugar breaks down into fructose and glucose. Complex carbohydrate (starch), however, breaks down only into glucose. This difference may have crucial implications.

The liver tissue of people with high blood fats incorporated fructose five times more rapidly than those with low blood fats. The fat tissue of people with high blood fats incorporated fructose seven to eight times more rapidly.

Why is this significant?

It points out again that people have different susceptibilities to the effect of eating sugar. One person will eat sugar with no effect on blood fats such as cholesterol and triglycerides. But another person, with a different biochemistry, will eat it and the sugar will raise those levels.

In susceptible individuals, the fat tissue rapidly takes up the fructose. Most of this fructose is quickly incorporated into fatty acids. A large percentage of these fatty acids are released into the bloodstream and then transported to the liver. The liver incorporates them into the triglycerides and then releases them as low-density lipoproteins (LDL).

High levels of triglycerides and LDL cholesterol (the "bad" cholesterol) are associated with increased risk of heart attack.

nervous system (SNS) activity, commonly known as the fight-or-flight response. The stimulatory effect has been shown to result from the sugar and fat content of their diets.

Other studies have confirmed that in animals and humans, simple carbohydrate administration increases SNS activity, and increased SNS activity promotes high blood pressure.

Sugar consumption has been statistically linked to atherosclerosis. Again, a link doesn't constitute proof. Yet researchers at the University of Pennsylvania may have found a partial explanation for this finding.

Fat, Frying, and Disease

Scientists are now uncovering mechanisms to explain the statistical links between fat consumption and cholesterol, heart disease, and cancer.

Fats and related substances are known as lipids. Lipids, particularly in the form of polyunsaturated fats, readily combine with oxygen in a process called oxidation. When lipids become loaded with oxygen, they are called peroxides, which:

- Can injure the walls of the arteries, which may lead to atherosclerosis and heart disease
- Can break DNA molecules and destroy the enzymes that normally repair broken DNA, which may lead to cancer
- Generate free radicals (highly reactive substances) that set off chain reactions by converting even more lipids into peroxides (the free radicals cause a snowballing reaction resulting in destruction of cell walls, enzyme systems, and essential biochemical processes)

Deep-fat frying is particularly dangerous because it promotes faster oxidation, peroxide formation, and free radical reactions.

Because polyunsaturated oils (liquid at room temperature) oxidize most quickly, frying with them is dangerous. Frying with saturated fats is even more dangerous because of its effect of raising blood cholesterol.

Oxidation is a problem not only with fried foods, but with many processed foods as well. Processed foods have been stripped of the vitamins and minerals that inhibit oxidation (see chapter 12). Additionally, processed foods, such as bleached flour, often contain readily oxidized additives and so may be more likely to form dangerous peroxides.

Prudent Action

Why not be cautious and sensible about fats in your diet, even though the fats/disease connection in humans is still being debated? We do know that:

- Diets high in polyunsaturated fats promote cancer in animals.
- A wealth of studies link high-fat diets to breast and other cancers. (It must also be noted that other studies fail to find these links.)
- Most physicians feel that high-fat diets are linked with high blood cholesterol. (Other physicians note that 90 percent of the blood cholesterol is synthesized by the liver and claim the effects of diet on cholesterol levels are exaggerated.)

What's the result? While conclusive proof may be lacking about the negative effects of sugar, fat, frying, and processing on disease, strongly suggestive evidence is available.

Based on this evidence, a prudent approach would dictate eliminating or limiting those substances and substituting foods that promote health (see chapter 12).

Questions Begging for Answers

"Okay," you say, "I want to be prudent, but . . .

"If I'm eating ⅕ to ⅓ pound of sugar a day, how do I know where to find it in order to eliminate it?"

"How do I handle my cravings for sweets?"

"What do I do if I'm unwilling to give up cakes, candies, cookies, and the like, but want to have optimal health and weight?"

"If my diet is 60 percent sugar and fat, what do I eat to replace it?"

"I know that some fat is essential. What fats should I eat and how much?"

"If I give up sugar, how do I stop myself from feeling like I'm on the Body-Signal Sugar-Deprivation Program?"

"The supermarkets only sell 'enriched' bread. Where do I find whole-grain alternatives?"

"If I want to give up sugar and artificial sweeteners, how do I sweeten my food and drinks without causing problems?"

The Body-Signal Program will answer these questions and teach you how to put everything you've learned into action.

Now that you've found that so many of your favorite foods are fraught with peril, you'll be happy to discover that lots of the other foods you love to eat will improve your health and ward off disease.

Chapter 12

Nutritional Signals

*Eating a health-promoting diet
really requires no great effort. Expand
your repertoire just a little bit and you can
deliciously taste your way to better health.*

Nutrition courses used to irritate me beyond measure. So did most nutrition books. Why? They rarely addressed what concerned me. Sure, they talked endlessly about vitamins, minerals, deficiency states, fiber, calories, carbohydrates, protein, amino acids, lipids—but they never talked about the main point: *Food!*

I wanted to know what I should be eating—and why. I wanted to know which foods would help prevent illness and promote health—and why. Basically, that's all I wanted to know.

"Leave all this other stuff to the research scientists," I'd tell myself. "I'm not interested."

Okay. I was a *bit* interested. I realized I *did* want to know about the science behind the nutritional findings—but not at the expense of real food information. Over the years, my patients and seminar participants have echoed that irritation. Their questions about food confirmed that while many of us may be interested in learning the latest research, *all* of us are interested in learning what foods to eat and what those foods do to and for our bodies.

How to Turn On Nutritional Signals

When it comes to knowing what to eat, I have three personal theories.

Theory 1: You don't need a nutritionist to tell you what to eat or how much to eat. All you have to do is tune into your own mental, emotional, and physical signals.

Theory 2: Given the fact that your taste experience comes from a diet that is 20 percent the taste of sugar, 40 percent the taste of fat, and who-knows-how-much the taste of artificial flavorings, it just may be that you've lost touch with the extremely satisfying experience of tasting the foods we'll discuss in this chapter.

Theory 3: When you switch from the standard American diet to a nutritious diet, you'll not only derive important health benefits, but you'll facilitate the loss of extra weight. Since you'll be reducing your intake of fat-promoting foods and increasing your intake of high-fiber, obesity-fighting foods, it makes sense.

If these theories are correct, here's what they mean.

- If you were to tune in to your taste for "real" food, you would know just what you want to eat.
- If you weren't in the mood for foods with sugar, fat, or artificial flavoring, you would know which foods would "hit the spot."
- If I simply provided you with some lists of so-called healthy foods, you would instinctively know which and how much of these foods you wanted to eat.
- With this selection of "healthy" foods, you would choose enough variety to provide you with all the nutrients necessary for optimal health.

That's exactly what is going to happen.

I'm going to provide you with lists of foods. But since this is a book and not a grocery list, I also feel compelled to offer you some studies that show just what make these foods truly good for you.

Food surveys have shown that most people eat the same 15 or 16 foods over and over again. If you're one of these people, don't let the expansive lists of foods you're about to see intimidate you.

Relax. Just settle back and let your mind begin to absorb the choices and variety of foods available to you. As you begin to recognize your nutritional signals, you'll know what you want to eat. You'll find that some of the "new" foods will not only satisfy your desire for savory, delicious dishes, but also could help to heal or prevent certain physical problems.

My purpose here is to expose you to this wide variety of health-promoting foods. The Body-Signal Program (see chapter 13) will teach you just how to introduce these foods into your repertoire.

The Four Big Food Questions

Along with learning which foods to eat and what these foods do to and for our bodies, there are certain specific questions most of us want to ask. Let's take a look at the four big ones.

1. Can nutritional changes prevent specific diseases or ailments?
2. What health problems are helped by what foods? How much of these foods should I eat and how often?
3. What components of these foods are considered health promoting?
4. What evidence is there to support these claims?

Now let's go for some answers.

Seven Critical Conditions

You want to know if nutritional changes can prevent specific diseases or conditions. Here's the answer: Apparently, they can.

Scientists are accumulating evidence that shows certain foods do have specific health-promoting properties. They find that eating ample quantities of these foods may increase your chances of warding off certain health problems. These problems include:

- Cancer
- Atherosclerosis (hardening of the arteries)
- High blood pressure and stroke
- High cholesterol
- High triglycerides (blood fats)
- Gastrointestinal problems
- Diabetes mellitus

And that's not all. While researchers have been collecting some fascinating data on health-promoting foods, some nutritionists have been much impressed by anecdotal reports (not verified by strict scientific study) from patients who claim a health problem has improved after a dietary change. These nutritionists also feel that certain medical conditions, osteoporosis for instance, can be prevented, or that the duration of the common cold can be shortened by improving the quality of what we eat. Like them, I've also been impressed by reports from my patients and seminar graduates who have told me, for example, that after making dietary changes, they've noticed an increase in their energy level or relief from their arthritic pains.

Some of these reports have been truly dramatic. And while I don't know if these claims are true, I do think that they're worthy of our consideration.

The Magic Ingredients

No, it's not all done with mirrors. There are actual substances in foods that promote good health. What are these substances?

- Insoluble fiber, including nondigestible fibers such as cellulose
- Soluble fiber, such as pectin and guar gum
- Vitamins, such as A, B-complex, C, D, E, and beta-carotene
- Macro-minerals (found in large quantities in your body), such as calcium, potassium, and magnesium
- Trace minerals, such as selenium and zinc

FOOD SUPPLEMENTS— OR THE REAL THING?

It has been shown that some ailments are helped by diets rich in certain foods—or aggravated by diets lacking certain foods (and/or nutrients). Also, some health problems have been relieved by nutrients taken in the form of supplements.

There's an important distinction here. If a nutrient is helpful as part of your food diet, there's no proof that the same nutrient administered as a supplement will be equally helpful. Conversely, if a supplement is seen to affect a health concern favorably—folate tablets and poor circulation, or vitamin C and the common cold, for example—that doesn't necessarily mean that a diet rich in folate or vitamin C will be equally beneficial.

Much of the information about the effect of supplements on diseases is very compelling—but also very controversial.

• Fish oils, such as omega-3 fatty acids
• Olive oil
• Amino acids (the building blocks of protein), such as methionine
• Lecithin
• Sulfur

Some of the "magic" of these ingredients comes from their antioxidant properties. Antioxidants control the body's free radicals—highly combustible molecular fragments that can harm cellular functioning and contribute to both degenerative diseases and the aging process. All of the vitamins and trace minerals on the above list are antioxidants.

Now let's take a look at the health problems that can be helped—and by which foods.

Cancer

Scan the list of cancer-fighting foods that follows on page 200, and get ready to talk food. Let's talk beans; let's talk bread; let's talk melons and tomatoes, strawberries and broccoli, brussels sprouts and cabbage, and onions and garlic! These are the real foods that apparently work to prevent cancer.

Fiber

Some nutrition scientists believe that if you promote speedy passage of foods through the intestinal tract, there will be less chance for intestinal toxins to accumulate. The result will be a lower risk of colon cancer. Dutch researchers have shown that the insoluble fiber of beans has just such an effect in pushing things along!

For this same reason, fiber-rich, whole-grain bread should also be on your list of cancer preventives. While working in Africa, famed British researcher Denis P. Burkitt noticed the rarity of colon cancer among Africans whose diet was high in fiber. He reported on his findings often and convincingly in the journals and in several books.

Vitamins A and C

Do you ever get a yen for a fruit like cantaloupe? If you do, go for it. Studies at the National Cancer Institute linked a good intake of melons to a lower incidence of esophageal cancer. Researchers at Harvard Medical School found the lowest cancer rates in people who ate similar

Cancer-Fighting Foods

Foods	Nutrient/Component
Beans and legumes Garbanzo beans (chick-peas), green beans, kidney beans, lima beans, navy beans, pinto beans, soybeans	Insoluble fiber and soluble fiber, such as guar gum
Fruit Cantaloupe, casaba melon, honeydew melon, strawberries, tomatoes, watermelon	Vitamins A and C
Allium vegetables Chives, garlic, leeks, onions, shallots	Sulfides
Cruciferous vegetables Bok choy, broccoli, brussels sprouts, cabbage, cauliflower	Indoles, vitamins A and C, calcium
Dark green vegetables Collard greens, kale, mustard greens, spring chard, turnip greens	Calcium, beta-carotene, and fiber
Red, yellow, and orange vegetables Butternut squash, carrots, sweet potatoes, yams, zucchini	Beta-carotene
Whole-grain products Buckwheat pancakes; cornbread; corn tortillas; five- or seven-grain bread; whole wheat bread, muffins, pita, or pretzels	Insoluble fiber

foods such as tomatoes or strawberries every week. It makes sense. These foods are good sources of vitamins A and C—*and* fiber.

The Cabbage Family

When you were a kid (and maybe even now), you probably didn't receive a whole lot of nutritional signals telling you to eat cabbage! This food was probably as popular with you as okra.

Yet it looks like the cabbage family (cruciferous vegetables) just may be a good disease preventive. As a matter of fact, when it comes to cancer, it may be the best.

Scientists are studying substances that detoxify chemicals in the body—"cancer inhibitors." Among these cancer inhibitors are indoles, which are found in cruciferous vegetables. One survey showed that people who rarely ate cabbage were three times more likely to get cancer than people who ate it at least once a week.

Broccoli: A perfect food. If you look for all these cancer inhibitors in one place—indoles, carotene, and vitamin C, plus calcium—you'll find them together in the most perfect cancer-preventing food: broccoli. A food survey of 1,000 men confirmed it—eating broccoli was associated with a lower risk of colon cancer. Another thing that makes broccoli a perfect food is that it's a very tasty vegetable!

Beta-Carotene

Believe it or not, many people who have kicked the sugar habit find they can satisfy their sweet tooth signals with certain vegetables. Carrots and sweet potatoes are two good examples: Both contain large amounts of beta-carotene.

Beta-carotene is the plant form of vitamin A, and it's a good example of a nutrient with antioxidant properties. Beta-carotene has been linked to decreased levels of cancer.

Carotene is abundant in red, orange, and yellow vegetables and in many fruits. The vitamin A in $\frac{1}{3}$ cup of cooked carrots or $\frac{1}{4}$ of a sweet potato eaten daily is the amount of vitamin A considered sufficient to reduce the incidence of cancer of the lung, esophagus, stomach, intestines, mouth, throat, larynx, bladder, and prostate—perhaps by as much as 50 percent.

Help for smokers. The high price smokers pay in terms of disease is all too well documented. But a simple thing like getting more beta-carotene can help turn the tide for them. The *Lancet,* Britain's leading medical journal, published a 19-year study in which 2,000 middle-aged men were monitored. The results are in the table on page 202.

Subjects	Death Rate (%)
Nonsmokers	16
Former smokers	20
Smokers—1 to 14 cigarettes a day	23
Smokers—15 to 24 cigarettes a day	30
Smokers—25+ cigarettes a day	35

There were 33 deaths due to lung cancer. Now look at these figures.

Beta-Carotene Intake of Subjects	Lung Cancer Rate (%)
Overall	
Lowest intake of beta-carotene	2.9
Highest intake of beta-carotene	0.4
Among men who smoked at least 30 years	
Lowest intake of beta-carotene	6.4
Highest intake of beta-carotene	0.8

This means that when 500 men with the highest intake of carotene were compared to 500 men with the lowest intake, there was seven times less lung cancer in the high-carotene group (2 men to 14).

The National Academy of Sciences and the National Cancer Institute have reported numerous studies that confirm the beneficial effect of vitamin A on cancer (and dozens more are in progress).

Example 1: A cancer researcher in Tucson, Arizona, gave a daily dose of beta-carotene equivalent to the amount found in ten carrots to 24 patients with leukoplakia (a precancerous mouth sore). After six months, 17 of the patients showed a marked reduction in the size of their mouth sores. Preliminary data suggest that the sores recur when beta-carotene is stopped.

Example 2: Research shows that vitamin A may help cervical cancer, which kills 7,000 women in America every year. Recent evidence indicates that women who eat diets high in vitamin A and/or beta-carotene may be less likely to develop cervical cancer.

Example 3: Cervical cancer is strongly suspected of being linked to a specific virus (HPV), which appears to turn normal cells into cancer cells. Doctors at the University of South Carolina School of Medicine found that vitamin A stops or dramatically slows the growth of HPV cells. Ongoing studies are aimed at finding out how this happens.

Example 4: A Japanese study correlates a high intake of vitamin A–rich yellow and green vegetables with a lower rate of prostate cancer.

More Antioxidants to Battle Cancer

Similar cancer-prevention traits show up in vitamins C and E and in selenium. For example:

* People in Northern France and China who ate diets low in vitamin C–rich fruits and vegetables had notably high rates of esophageal cancer.
* Researchers at Albert Einstein College of Medicine in New York have correlated low vitamin C intake with cervical cancer.
* Formation of intestinal mutagens (substances found in the intestinal tract that could cause gene damage and possibly trigger cancer) was reduced by supplementation with vitamins C and E.
* When the trace mineral selenium was added to drinking water, it helped protect test animals from cancer-causing chemicals.

Excellent sources of vitamin C include the fruits and vegetables cited in "Cancer-Fighting Foods" on page 200, plus sprouted alfalfa seeds, acerola cherries, citrus fruits, rose hips, and green peppers.

Sources of vitamin E include cold-pressed vegetable oils, wheat germ, eggs, organ meats, sweet potatoes, leafy vegetables, whole grains, and nuts.

The selenium content of food depends largely on the soil in which the food is grown. For this reason, it's often difficult to judge how much selenium we're getting in our diets. But for your best shot, look to grain products including wheat germ and bran, sesame seeds, brewer's yeast, tuna, and herring.

Sulfides: Special Agents

Another set of substances that may act as antioxidant, anti-cancer agents contain sulfur. You may have to sacrifice sweet breath for good health, but if your antenna is signaling for onions and garlic, the sacrifice is worthwhile. Two examples of sulfur-containing agents are sulfides—found in onions, garlic, and other allium vegetables—and glutathione—a compound occurring naturally in some foods, which may include onions and garlic as well as other vegetables.

Researchers in China who surveyed 685 patients with stomach cancer made a fascinating discovery in the process. They found that they all had one curious thing in common—they all ate less than 25 pounds of allium vegetables a year. To find out if this phenomenon actually meant anything, the scientists looked at 1,131 people who did not have stomach cancer and found that these people ate 25 to 50 pounds a year. As the consumption of allium vegetables increased, the risk of stomach cancer appeared to decrease.

Calcium and Vitamin D

It's not likely that your body will signal you to take a trip to Florida. But if it does, you might have a good nutritional reason for heeding its message. Here's why.

Vitamin D, which aids in the absorption of calcium, is produced by the body when it is exposed to sunlight. The calcium/vitamin D combination provides an example of a mineral and vitamin that apparently work together to reduce cancer risk. A strong link has been found between high calcium intake and a lower incidence of colon cancer. The vitamin D/calcium/colon cancer link provides a possible explanation for the lower incidence of colon cancer among New Yorkers who retire to Florida, compared with those who remain in the North.

For those who live in Norway, Lapland, or Antarctica and have minimal exposure to sunlight, there are other sources of vitamin D: salmon, sardines, herring, vitamin D–fortified milk and milk products, egg yolks, and organ meats.

Atherosclerosis

Diet has made its mark as a major player in the prevention and treatment of atherosclerosis and other circulation problems. A look at the list below will show you that many foods may have a pivotal role in prevention.

New reports of the effectiveness of diet appear in medical journals with reassuring regularity, and many researchers agree that a few simple changes in what you eat could protect you from these health threats.

Foods That Fight Atherosclerosis

Foods	Nutrient/Component
Beans and legumes Garbanzo beans (chick-peas), Great Northern beans, green beans, kidney beans, lentils, lima beans, navy beans, soybeans	Magnesium, vitamin B_6, and fiber (*Note:* Kidney beans, lima beans, and soybeans are some of the best legumes for B_6 and magnesium.)

Foods	Nutrient/Component
Deep-sea fish Anchovies, bluefish, herring, mackerel, sablefish, salmon, striped bass, swordfish	Fish oil and magnesium (*Note:* Salmon is also good for vitamin B_6, as is tuna to a lesser extent.)
Seafood Mussels, oysters, shrimp, squid	Fish oil
Fruit Avocado; banana; blackberries; boysenberries; cantaloupe; dates; grapefruit; loganberries; melons; oranges; peaches, dried; pears, dried; pineapple; plantains; prickly pears; prunes; raisins	Magnesium and fiber
Low-fat meats, poultry, and organ meats Beef, chicken breast, lamb, liver, pheasant, quail, turkey, veal	Vitamin B_6
Cruciferous vegetables Bok choy, broccoli, brussels sprouts, cabbage, cauliflower	Magnesium, vitamin B_6, and fiber
Vegetables Carrots, corn, peas, potatoes, spinach	Vitamin B_6
Whole grains and whole-grain products Brown rice; buckwheat; buckwheat pancakes; bulgur; cornmeal and cornbread; corn tortillas; five- or seven-grain bread; groats; kasha; millet; pearled barley; rye flour; whole wheat bread, muffins, noodles, pita, or pretzels	Magnesium, vitamin B_6, and fiber

Atherosclerosis, B_6, and Monkey Business

If you're not in the mood to listen to your own signals, you might want to listen to some monkey signals. If you do, you're going to start eating a lot of foods rich in vitamin B_6. When that happens, you may be reducing your risk of atherosclerosis and heart attack significantly.

Let's listen to the monkeys—three different groups of them.

- The first group was fed a diet deficient in vitamin B_6. These monkeys rapidly developed atherosclerosis.
- The second group of monkeys had vitamin B_6 added to their diets. They wound up with lower cholesterol levels (and as you know, lower cholesterol levels are linked to a lower incidence of atherosclerosis).
- The third group was fed a diet high in cholesterol but also high in vitamin B_6. The vitamin B_6 allowed these monkeys to dispose of the extra cholesterol and thus maintain low serum cholesterol levels.

B_6, tryptophan, and your heart. The amino acid tryptophan is an important nutrient that has other functions besides putting people to sleep. (Many people have been taking it as a supplement to induce· sleep. However, in 1989, it was linked to over 500 cases of a rare blood disorder and at least one death.)

Tryptophan—an essential component of proteins—won't hurt you when you get it through food. But if you don't take in enough vitamin B_6, tryptophan won't metabolize properly. Instead, it forms a substance called xanthurenic acid.

What does your body do with the xanthurenic acid? It gets rid of it in urine. To measure xanthurenic acid levels in the urine, a group of cardiac patients was given tryptophan. Their levels of xanthurenic acid proved to be high, which meant they were getting too little vitamin B_6 to prevent the conversion of tryptophan to xanthurenic acid. This suggests that vitamin B_6 deficiency might be common among cardiac patients and may even be a causative factor in heart disease.

B_6 to beat fats. Cardiac patients aren't the only ones who excrete a lot of xanthurenic acid. Studies in Japan demonstrate that people who eat high-fat diets also excrete more of the acid. What's interesting here, according to those studies, is that the consumption of extra fat evidently promotes vitamin B_6 deficiency.

So what do we need? Less fat or more vitamin B_6? Probably both.

Again, let's listen to the monkeys. Some monkey studies have shown that high levels of B_6 protect against the effects of a high-fat, high-cholesterol diet.

Here's what you need to know. Although practically everyone claims you should worry about high-fat diets, that may only be a part of the story. It may be that a high-fat diet becomes more dangerous when it's combined with a low-B_6 diet.

Legumes

The complex carbohydrates of leguminous seeds (beans, lentils, split peas, peanuts) have a cholesterol-lowering action. Their B_6 and fiber content may account for part of the reason.

Vitamin C and Magnesium

When vitamin C was given to animals with high cholesterol levels, it lowered their levels and reduced the extent and severity of their atherosclerosis. Similarly, rats fed diets that ordinarily produce atherosclerosis were protected when their magnesium consumption was increased.

More Fiber!

The "Boston Brothers Study" has been sponsored by the Harvard School of Public Health for 30 years. In this study, researchers monitored the diets and health of 500 men born in Ireland (who emigrated to Boston) and their brothers (who remained in Ireland). Most of the 150 men who died of heart disease over this 30-year period shared a particular habit—they ate low-fiber diets short on grains and vegetable proteins.

A Little Fish Story

Certain deep-sea fish contain omega-3 fatty acids, a fish-oil substance that protects against heart disease. Two to three servings a week may be all that's required to ward off heart attacks!

High Blood Pressure and Stroke

Fish oils do more than prevent heart attacks. They're also being studied as a blood pressure–lowering agent. And, as the following list illustrates, many foods just as commonplace as fish provide a protective shield against one of the most threatening health problems of modern times.

Defenders against High Blood Pressure and Stroke

Foods	Nutrient/Component
Beans and legumes Black beans, black-eyed peas, garbanzo beans (chick-peas), Great Northern beans, green beans, kidney beans, lentils, lima beans, navy beans, soybeans, split peas, tofu	Potassium and calcium
Deep-sea fish Anchovies, bluefish, herring, mackerel, sablefish, salmon, striped bass, swordfish	Potassium, calcium, and fish oil (*Note:* Sardines, salmon, and mackerel are good sources of calcium. Cod, halibut, salmon, scallops, snapper, and tuna are good sources of potassium.)
Fruit Apricots, dried; avocado; bananas; cantaloupe; dates; figs, dried; oranges; papaya; peaches, dried; pears, dried; plantains; prunes; raisins	Potassium
Low-fat meats, poultry, and organ meats Beef, chicken breast, goose, lamb, liver, pheasant, quail, turkey, veal	Potassium
Milk and yogurt	Calcium
Nuts and seeds Almonds, brazil nuts, hazelnuts, sesame and sunflower seeds, tahini (sesame-seed paste)	Calcium
Japanese seaweeds Agar-agar, hiziki, kelp, kombu, nori, wakami	Calcium

Foods	Nutrient/Component
Dark green vegetables Beet greens, collard greens, kale, mustard greens, spring chard, turnip greens	Calcium
Vegetables Carrots, okra, parsley, parsnips, potatoes, pumpkin, tomatoes, winter squash, yams	Potassium and calcium

Calcium

Believe it or not, it may even turn out that it's a good health practice to listen to your mother's nutritional signals! After all, she's the one who told you to drink your milk, right?

Milk is another food that may have a beneficial effect on blood pressure. A survey in Puerto Rico of 8,000 men showed that those who didn't drink milk were twice as likely to have high blood pressures as those who drank at least a quart a day.

To determine if it was the calcium content of milk that produced this effect, a group of several hundred Americans was given milk fortified with extra calcium. In this group, blood pressures dropped an average of 6 to 7 points.

However, many nutritionists feel the hazards of milk outweigh the benefits. Their objections include:

• The fat content
• The potential for idiosyncratic or allergic reactions
• Gastrointestinal upset due to lactose intolerance (an inability to metabolize milk sugar)
• The potential for osteoporosis due to the high phosphorus content of milk (see "The Osteoporosis/Calcium Controversy" on page 221).

If you want to look elsewhere for calcium, look to seaweeds—the richest source. The Japanese eat seaweeds the way we eat salads. But if you just can't seem to develop a taste for this "new" food (in other words, if the idea of eating seaweed makes you go "Ugh!"), don't worry. Dark green vegetables such as those in the cabbage family, particularly bok choy and collard greens, are full of calcium. Two servings a day should be your minimum. As the above list shows, the array of calcium-rich foods is vast enough to suit anyone's taste.

Potassium

Another macro-mineral that's demonstrating a positive impact on health is potassium. A Japanese study compared two villages whose inhabitants showed a dramatic difference in blood pressures. The village inhabitants with the lower pressures had higher levels of potassium intake.

A diet loaded with potassium also appears to protect against strokes. In a 12-year study conducted at the University of California on almost 900 men, those with the lowest potassium intake suffered 2½ to 4 times more strokes than those with higher potassium intake.

Is Vegetarianism for You?

I think becoming a vegetarian should be an individual choice. But if you have high blood pressure, you may want to consider it as a therapeutic measure. There's a good reason: Vegetables have less saturated fat than meat and contain more polyunsaturated fat. This might be the explanation for the drop in blood pressure that was observed in high blood pressure subjects who were switched to meat-free diets.

High Cholesterol and Triglycerides

Fish, along with numerous other foods, is considered to be beneficial in cutting high cholesterol and triglyceride levels. Check out the table on page 212 for examples of the variety of foods that may ensure arterial health.

Fish-Oil Findings

In 1985, the *New England Journal of Medicine* reported that fish oil lowers cholesterol and triglycerides. A diet rich in salmon oil was found to lower cholesterol by as much as 20 percent and triglycerides 40 to 60 percent. Studies in Japan showed the highest HDL ("good") cholesterol levels in those people who ate the most fish.

Studies around the world confirm the effect of fish oil on triglycerides. For example, East African tribesmen who ate a lot of fish had an average triglyceride level 31 percent lower than those tribesmen who didn't eat fish.

Olive Oil

Another oil that has a beneficial effect on cholesterol is olive oil. Unlike other oils, which may lower HDL and LDL ("bad") cholesterol, olive oil appears to lower only LDL cholesterol. Look for bottles marked "E.V.C.P."—extra virgin cold pressed (not cold processed!). It comes from the first pressing.

Fat Busters

Wouldn't it be great if you could eat foods that would dissolve the fat in your bloodstream? You can!

When there is more lecithin in the blood than cholesterol, there is less tendency for fat deposits to form in blood vessels. For instance, in one study, animals were fed diets with excessive cholesterol but adequate lecithin. They did *not* develop atherosclerosis. That's what you call fat busting.

Note: Foods that contain lecithin may also be beneficial in lowering cholesterol. Some sources include corn, liver, nuts, soybeans, whole wheat, and unrefined vegetable oils. Although eggs also contain lecithin, they should not be considered a means of lowering serum cholesterol.

Nutrients such as methionine (an amino acid) and B vitamins choline and inositol aid the body's production of lecithin (as do vitamin B_6 and magnesium). In a Harvard study, monkeys fed a diet that was adequate in every way except for methionine deficiency did develop atherosclerosis.

Conversely, animals who were fed an atherogenic diet (a diet designed to *foster* atherosclerosis) but supplemented with methionine showed no atherosclerosis or elevated cholesterol levels. In other words, scientists had to combine a diet high in fat and cholesterol with a diet deficient in methionine to produce elevated serum cholesterol and atherosclerosis. Again, that's what you call fat busting.

In another study, 115 out of 230 heart patients were given extra choline. At the end of three years, only 12 of the men given the choline had died, while 30 of the men who did *not* receive choline were dead. More fat busting?

The beat goes on. Lecithin synthesis in rats is three times as high when both choline and cholesterol are part of their diets as opposed to rats on diets with only cholesterol. For this reason, when adequate choline is added to the meals of rats on high-fat, high-cholesterol diets, it's difficult to produce atherosclerosis experimentally.

Eating to Ease Elevated Cholesterol and/or Triglyceride Levels

Foods	Nutrient/Component
Beans and legumes Black beans, black-eyed peas, garbanzo beans (chick-peas), Great Northern beans, green beans, kidney beans, lentils, lima beans, navy beans, soybeans, split peas	Choline and fiber (*Note:* Soybeans are a rich source of choline.)
Deep-sea fish and seafood Anchovies, bluefish, herring, sablefish, salmon, shark, snails, snapper, striped bass, swordfish, trout, tuna (packed in water)	Fish oil, choline, and methionine
Fruits Avocado; banana; blackberries; boysenberries; cantaloupe; dates; grapefruit; loganberries; melon; oranges; peaches, dried; pears, dried; pineapples; plantains; prickly pears; prunes; raisins	Magnesium, fiber
Nuts and seeds Brazil nuts, pumpkin seeds, sesame seeds, squash seeds, sunflower seeds	Methionine and inositol
Olive oil	Monounsaturated fat
Organ meats Beef liver, calves' liver, chicken livers, kidneys	Choline

Foods	Nutrient/Component
Poultry Chicken, duck, pheasant, quail, turkey	Methionine
Cruciferous vegetables Bok choy, broccoli, brussels sprouts, cabbage, cauliflower	Fiber, including pectin
Vegetables Carrots, corn, peas, potatoes, spinach	Vitamin B_6
Whole grains and whole-grain products Brown rice; buckwheat; buckwheat pancakes; bulgur; cornmeal and cornbread; corn tortillas; five- or seven-grain bread; groats; kasha; millet; pearled barley; rye flour; whole wheat bread, muffins, noodles, pita, or pretzels	Magnesium, vitamin B_6, fiber

A Low-Cholesterol Menu: An Overrated Idea?

Cut down on dietary cholesterol. Is this an overrated idea? Maybe.

If you lower your *serum* cholesterol, you lower your chance of a heart attack. Given that premise, logic dictates that if you lower your *dietary* cholesterol, your *serum* cholesterol should also fall. This sounds good, but it just might not be true.

About 90 percent of serum cholesterol comes from the liver. When dietary cholesterol is increased, the liver tends to lower its serum cholesterol production. If you have a high cholesterol level and go on a low-cholesterol diet to reduce it, the liver's balancing act might just prevent you from obtaining the results you want.

This means that the first line of defense against high cholesterol may *not* be a low-cholesterol diet. Next to listening to your Body Signals, the first line of defense may be a diet rich in foods that contain lecithin, methionine, choline, inositol, vitamin B_6, and magnesium.

With this in mind, it's not surprising that including food such as deep-sea fish, nuts, seeds, poultry, and legumes in your dietary repertoire may be good for your blood vessels.

"Fat busters! Who you gonna call? Lecithin!"

Some Cholesterol Surprises

Butter may be good for your cholesterol. And whole milk may be better than low-fat milk.

Heresy, you say? Let's take a look, and then let's take another look at something else—fat!

It seems that there were two credos for the 1980s—"Get fat and die" and "Eat fat and die." In chapter 10, you learned the truth about the first credo; now here's the truth about the second.

It isn't dangerous to eat fat. The problem is that the typical Western diet contains twice as much fat as it should. In other words, most nutritionists would agree that if you reduce your fat intake from 40 percent of your diet to 20 percent, you won't have fat-related nutritional problems. Pritikin is the only major voice who disagrees, claiming that fat content should be reduced to 10 percent of your intake. If you can eat that little fat without developing an antipathy toward food, then more power to you.

Most of us aren't aware of the fat content of the foods we eat. For instance, a regular muffin can contain as much as 40 percent fat. Croissants are the same. This means that most of the fat you eat is "hidden" in processed foods and junk foods. If you cut down on these foods, then you're not likely to get into trouble by eating butter and eggs and drinking milk.

The calcium/fat connection. Animal studies show that in order to absorb enough of the calcium that we ingest, we need to eat sufficient fat. The absorption of dietary calcium requires the presence of sufficient fat, but if we eat too much fat, calcium absorption is depressed.

Butterfat permits calcium absorption. (It also augments the growth of intestinal flora that produce vitamin B_6. Do you recall the beneficial effect of B_6 on atherosclerosis?)

What does this have to do with cholesterol?

Calcium works to keep serum cholesterol at normal levels. How this happens isn't clear. (Perhaps it's due to increased excretion of fat and of bile acids that form cholesterol.) The result, however, is that calcium has a protective action against atherosclerosis.

Example 1: Increased calcium intake in young men and women has been shown to cause a significant reduction in serum cholesterol and triglycerides.

Example 2: Southern Madras Indians eat a diet containing 2 percent saturated fat. The fat content in the diet of Northern Indians is 19 times greater—they eat a lot of butterfat and fermented milk drinks. Contrary to what you'd expect, the heart disease rate of the Northern Indians was 15 times lower.

The "whole" (milk) thing? If you're going to drink milk and you want to spare your cholesterol, the milk had better be lowfat. Good advice? Probably not.

Interestingly, since butterfat is essential to calcium absorption, and calcium deficiency may contribute to atherosclerosis, whole milk may be better for maintaining a safe cholesterol level than low-fat milk.

What does this mean to you?

It means that if you like milk, you can now drink it knowing that it may help your blood pressure and your cholesterol.

A good word about eggs. In some ways, eggs are close to being the most perfect of foods. Few foods are as rich in vitamins and minerals as eggs. Eggs include antioxidant nutrients, including the sulfur-containing amino acids that are not readily available in many of the foods we eat. Eggs even contain some of the fat busters, such as lecithin.

The questions arise: Do we eat eggs for their great nutritional value? Or do we avoid eggs—limiting ourselves to a maximum of four a week as the American Heart Association suggests—to protect our cholesterol levels?

My decision is influenced by studies done by animal investigators. They found that while eggs did raise cholesterol levels, there was no increase in arterial lesions, atherosclerosis, morbidity, and the shortening of life—presumably due to lecithin. In fact, the animals who ate eggs daily lived the longest. Similarly, with few exceptions, humans who participated in studies where eggs or egg yolks were consumed in large quantities did not develop elevated cholesterol levels.

A personal note. Am I advocating butter, whole milk, and eggs as part of a cholesterol-lowering regimen? *Your* cholesterol-lowering regimen?

No.

I am making the important point that there is no reason to fear healthful foods.

I eat a lot of butter because I like its taste. On occasion, I pour milk on my cereal. Some weeks I eat no eggs and other weeks I eat a few more than the American Heart Association recommends.

Yet because I eat so few processed foods, occasional cheeses, no fried foods, and moderate amounts of red meat, I know there's no way that I, personally, can consume enough dairy products to harm myself. In fact, given butter's effect on calcium absorption and its stimulation of B_6 in the intestine, eating butter probably benefits my health. The same could be said of eggs.

Isn't it mind-boggling to think that a *moderate* amount of dairy products ingested in the framework of a low-fat diet may actually promote good health rather than damage it?

How Fiber Fights High Cholesterol

Eating beans that contain a soluble fiber called guar gum has been shown to lower cholesterol levels. And pectin, another soluble fiber, has also been shown to be beneficial. Pectin is found in many fruits (apples, apricots, bananas, figs, and prunes), cruciferous vegetables, greens, beans, oat bran, oatmeal, and potatoes. Pectin is a somewhat less dramatically effective cholesterol-lowering agent than guar gum. Still, four to six daily servings of pectin-rich foods should help to lower your serum cholesterol.

James Anderson, M.D., who has gained fame for his work on dietary fiber at the University of Kentucky, reports:

• Thirty percent reductions in blood cholesterol levels on a high-fiber diet
• A 19 percent cholesterol level reduction on a diet containing the equivalent of a cup of cooked dry beans a day.

When other researchers replaced sugars, breads, and potatoes with split peas, lima beans, and common beans such as kidney beans, they saw a 9 percent drop in cholesterol levels. And in Holland, researchers found that a high intake of beans produced a significant drop in cholesterol levels.

Soybeans provide a double whammy against cholesterol. It's not surprising. Soybeans are rich in soluble fiber, calcium, and potassium.

Garbanzo beans (chick-peas) are another legume that should be part of every cholesterol-lowering regimen. A study in India substituted chick-peas for dietary wheat and cereals. The gratifying result was an average drop of 56 milligrams in cholesterol levels.

This is not to say that beans are better than grains in a cholesterol-lowering regimen. In another experimental diet, half the food intake was bread. The result was a 12 to 20 percent blood cholesterol reduction.

Many nutritionists feel that the daily intake of fiber should be 25 to 35 grams.

Oat bran overrated as a cholesterol cutter. Oat bran has had a great deal of attention lately as a food that lowers high cholesterol levels. But you really have to eat a lot of it to produce dramatic results. Before you buy your oat bran products, there are two cautions: (1) Read the label on your oat bran muffins—quite often, the second ingredient is sugar; and (2) don't depend on a little oat bran alone to lower cholesterol. Do provide yourself with a diet that includes oat bran along with all the cholesterol-lowering foods.

Some of Dr. Anderson's subjects ate the equivalent of two large oat bran muffins every day. They lowered their cholesterol level by almost 10 percent.

Another group of Dr. Anderson's subjects ate oat bran in amounts that exceeded a cup a day (contained in hot cereal and five muffins). These men, all of whom had a high cholesterol level, lowered their individual levels by 20 percent.

You can see that if you were going to depend on oat bran alone to cut your cholesterol count, you'd practically have to force-feed yourself to get it all in.

Gastrointestinal Diseases

Hold the Ex-Lax. Reach for fiber: wheat bran, oat bran, rye meal. They've all been shown to relieve constipation. In one study, patients who increased their consumption of these foods decreased their intake of laxatives by 93 percent.

In another study, patients switched from white bread to whole wheat and reported improved digestion. For patients with irritable bowel syndrome (IBS), this is especially important. When IBS patients switched to a diet high in insoluble wheat fiber, they reported less pain. Further, in half the IBS patients, bowel habits improved.

Irritable bowel syndrome isn't the only condition helped by cook-

Foods That Battle Bowel Problems

Foods	Nutrient/Component
Whole grains and whole-grain products Oat bran; rye meal; wheat bran; whole wheat bread, muffins, or pretzels	Fiber

ing with wheat bran. Researchers in one study gave patients with diverticular disease (a painful digestive disorder) 2 teaspoons of wheat bran a day. The results? Ninety percent reported dramatic improvement.

As a matter of fact, dietary histories reveal that high-fiber diets may actually prevent diverticular disease. It's been shown that people who eat a lot of meat and few vegetables are 50 percent more likely to suffer from diverticulosis than those who eat a little meat and a lot of vegetables.

Some nutritionists also think fiber plays a role in preventing hiatal hernia. Populations that eat high fiber or vegetarian diets are less likely to develop this condition.

Diabetes Mellitus

Dr. Anderson's work was originally aimed toward aiding diabetics. By placing his patients on a diet of high-fiber foods—beans, whole grains, and vegetables—he demonstrated impressive reductions in average levels of blood sugar. Many patients were able to stop taking their pills or insulin injections. And as a bonus, their triglyceride levels dropped by 15 percent.

High-fiber meals have more of a restraining effect on insulin levels when compared with low-fiber meals. The high fiber helps to balance out diabetics, who can show wide fluctuations in insulin levels between the fed and fasted state. See the table on the opposite page for foods that help stabilize diabetes mellitus.

Nutritional Controversies

Football fans fight about the value of "instant replay," and our art critics wrangle over Warhol's contribution. What gets nutritionists up and yelling? Vitamin C versus colds and the role of dietary calcium in osteoporosis.

The Common Cold Controversy

Does vitamin C prevent colds? I doubt it. But according to some researchers, it does make the symptoms slightly less severe, and it short-

Eating to Stabilize Diabetes Mellitus

Foods	Nutrient/Component
Beans and legumes Garbanzo beans (chick-peas), green beans, kidney beans, lima beans, navy beans, pinto beans, soybeans	Fiber
Cruciferous vegetables Bok choy, broccoli, brussels sprouts, cabbage, cauliflower	Fiber
Whole grains and whole-grain products Brown rice; buckwheat; buckwheat pancakes; bulgur; cornmeal and cornbread; corn tortillas; five- or seven-grain bread; groats; kasha; millet; pearled barley; rye flour; whole wheat bread, muffins, noodles, pita, or pretzels	Fiber

ens their duration. This mild benefit was achieved experimentally with a daily dose of 250 milligrams of vitamin C, or about the amount contained in two 8-ounce glasses of orange juice.

For many years, I've been telling my patients with colds to suck on a zinc lozenge every hour. According to a *Consumer Reports* publication, I've been misleading them. Well, I don't think that's exactly true. I told my patients that some reports showed that sucking on a zinc lozenge every hour would decrease the duration of a cold and that other reports dispute these findings. Now I know that zinc lozenges used in this way are harmless, at worst. Basically, this is what's called practicing the "art" of medicine.

Actually, the best thing you can do for yourself when you get a cold is to "steam your head." You can boil a pot of water, remove it from the heat source, place a towel over your head, lean over the hot pot (be careful!) two or three times a day, and breathe in the steam or

A NOTE ABOUT FIBER

A report published in *Progress in Food and Nutrition Science* sums up the properties of fiber and notes that the second half of this century has witnessed the booming growth of a major technology—food engineering. According to the report, food engineers have achieved "technological advances [that] have reduced and refined man's plant food intake and consequently brought about an unprecedented decline in his consumption of dietary fiber."

We have learned about the effects of dietary fiber by observing the diseases that have emerged since the onset of the new food engineering.

Dietary fiber affects the function of our gastrointestinal tracts from one end to the other because it:

• Restricts caloric intake
• Slows gastric and small intestinal transit (perhaps allowing one to feel satiated with less food)
• Holds water, which increases fecal weight and pushes materials along (allowing less time for cancer-promoting toxins to accumulate)
• Influences the release of gastrointestinal hormones
• Supports healthy bacterial growth

In addition to its gastrointestinal effects, dietary fiber also prevents major changes in blood sugar after you eat, which in turn improves glucose tolerance. And fiber also has positive long-term effects on lipoprotein (lipid-protein molecules such as cholesterol) metabolism.

What does this mean to you?

It means that eating 25 to 35 grams of fiber a day may diminish your chances of suffering from the following health problems.

• Atherosclerosis
• Cholesterol gallstones
• Colorectal cancer

• Constipation
• Diabetes mellitus
• Diverticulosis

And one other—obesity.

As other reports have noted, since dietary fiber "dampens" the insulin fluctuations between eating and fasting, allows fat to be broken down, and effects the Satisfaction Signal, these actions "might tend to prevent obesity."

you can turn your bathroom into a steam room and sit in it for 20 minutes before you go to bed. There's evidence that doing this will actually decrease the duration of your cold.

Since we've moved (for the moment) from real food to supplements, remember that even if vitamin C and zinc supplements do help colds, it doesn't mean that eating foods rich in these nutrients has the same effect. Sometimes supplements may be better "medicine" than food.

The Osteoporosis/Calcium Controversy

Some scientists point to inadequate calcium intake as the major problem. Some nutritionists point to certain foods and drinks that "drain" calcium. It's no wonder that the role of nutrition in osteoporosis is still unclear.

When animal and human subjects were fed foods containing more than twice as much phosphorus as calcium, something interesting occurred. The subjects began excreting calcium in their urine. Since blood calcium remains stable, presumably these subjects were losing calcium from their bones.

Again, what does this mean for you? That milk and soft drinks (beverages rich in phosphorus) are the worst offenders. It's ironic to think that the milk you're drinking specifically to make strong bones actually may be softening them!

Some nutritionists also claim that protein-dense foods (meat, for example) and foods that may affect acid-base balance could also be harmful. There is no firm evidence to support this notion. Nonetheless, according to this group of nutritionists, if you want to play it safe, you should avoid sugar, tobacco, wine and other alcoholic beverages, vinegar, citrus, caffeine, tea with lemon, and salt.

Are these recommendations valid for preventing osteoporosis? I don't know.

I do suggest that you eat the calcium-rich foods you've learned about and perhaps begin doing some weight-bearing exercises (push-ups, pull-ups, Nautilus or other weight training) on a regular basis.

Variety—The Spice of Health

By now, you know that there are numerous "new" foods that you can begin to experiment with and add to your meal repertoire.

What is the benefit of variety in the foods you eat? You're able to engage in worry-free eating. A varied diet means you don't have to plague yourself with those same meddlesome questions: "Did I eat enough potassium-rich foods today?" "Did I take in enough beta-carotene?"

Instead, you can pleasure yourself with these questions: "Which fruit (vegetables, grains, beans) am I in the mood for right now?" "How much do I feel like eating?" "What luxury foods (not-so-healthy foods that you love) do I want today?"

This is how you tune into your nutritional signals. Once you feel comfortable with the variety, your food propensities will change. You may find yourself:

- Eating some foods over and over again. Why? Because you just plain like them!
- Replacing some foods that you tend to eat repeatedly with other foods in the same category. Why? Because if you love baked beans, for example, and they're a constant source of culinary satisfaction, you may find yourself equally satisfied with lima beans, navy beans, and garbanzo beans.
- Eating some foods only occasionally. Why? Because your repertoire has expanded and you have more choices.
- Indulging occasionally in foods from the "bad" food categories—foods with sugar or refined flour or with a high fat content. But since you'll now know that you're eating a varied diet of primarily health-promoting foods, you'll be able to relax. Why? Because those small quantities of "bad" foods are not likely to harm you.

Variety is your key. It will open the door to the health-promoting "magic" substances, it will help you to tune in to your nutritional signals, and it will let you "taste" your way to good health in a most delicious fashion.

Chapter 13

The Six-Week Body-Signal Program

Transform your knowledge into success
by following this distillation
of the important lessons that lead to
Instinctive Eating for six weeks—and for life!

It's decision time!

You're now armed with a wealth of information—from your Body Signals and the Diet Mentality to the Instinctive Eater's mindset. You've also got a handle on self-acceptance, entitlement, body image, exercise, stress reduction, nutrition, making choices, getting what you want, and a lot more!

You will never be the same!

Even if you decide to toss this book on a shelf and take no action— you'll still never be the same. *You can't unlearn new awareness!*

At this point, there are two approaches you can take to put that awareness into action.

Approach 1: Mud against the Wall

Going on the premise that you *do* want to utilize what you've learned here, you could take action by using only those ideas that stick in your consciousness. Like throwing mud against the wall, whatever sticks, sticks. Whatever falls by the wayside, so be it.

It's a perfectly valid approach. And if you're willing to change, you will. However, the degree of change will depend on what you remember and what you put into practice.

Approach 2: Guaranteed Success— The Body-Signal Program

Simply finishing the book and waiting to "see" how things turn out is one way to go. But you do have an alternative that guarantees success: the Six-Week Body-Signal Program.

Here's what will happen. After you've completed the six weeks, you will have used the weight-control information, the behavioral illustrations, and the nutritional research to develop a dynamic new way of life. You'll have every tool you'll need to think, feel, and behave like a confident, self-caring human being *with no weight problem.* Will you have any regrets? Probably one. You'll wonder why you waited so long to get started!

Before You Begin...

As you continue reading, start thinking of a person or group that you'd like to enlist as your support station. (It may help to flip to "Back to the Future" on page 116 and review the role the support person plays.) Selecting an individual or team to report to concerning your progress will help you stay focused on producing results.

With support, you can't fail! If you can resist the impulse to act as a "Lone Ranger" in making your changes, *you'll have to succeed!*

Putting Knowledge into Action

Now that we're past the important preliminaries, what do you do on a day-to-day basis to solve your "weight problem" once and for all? Begin the Six-Week Body-Signal Program—*now.*

Here's what will happen. You'll be able to manage:

• Your Hunger Signals

- Your Satisfaction Signals
- Sugar, fat, alcohol, "enriched" white flour, fried foods, artificial sweeteners
- Exercise

And you'll learn how to:

- Get rid of the Diet Mentality
- Accept yourself and make peace with your appearance
- Feel entitled to fulfillment and high self-esteem
- Effectively deal with others *without* losing authority or feeling that you must apologize for yourself
- Do what you say you're going to do
- Manage stress

OVEREATERS ANONYMOUS

Overeaters Anonymous (OA) is the largest and most famous support group for victims of the Diet Mentality. The strength of this organization is demonstrated by its intense member support. People who attend OA meetings encourage each other to feel good about themselves, to take control of their lives, to eat nutritiously, and even to avoid diets. These are extremely important functions, and I can't applaud OA enough for creating this environment of understanding.

At the same time, if you're thinking of OA as a support alternative, you'd do well to consider one caveat. Every OA member who has ever attended my Lighten Up seminar has walked in clutching a negative label. "I have an addictive personality," one says. "I'm obsessive," says another. Still others declare, "I'm compulsive" or "I'm obsessive/compulsive" or "I have a personality problem that makes me crave instant gratification."

I'm against these labels. And there is good reason. It's been demonstrated over and over again that OA members are no different from any other seminar participant. Not one of them was ever taught to think like an Instinctive Eater and to respond to her Body Signals prior to attending the seminar.

For those of you currently attending OA meetings or planning to attend, please be aware that any OA participant who puts the Body-Signal Program into action will discover she has no need for disparaging labels. She is a *normal person* successfully managing her difficulties with food, weight, and self-image.

THE KEYS TO STRESS MANAGEMENT

1. Experience your emotions, whether pleasant or unpleasant.
2. Take control of what is within your control.
3. Accept (peacefully) what is not within your control.

Many people feel they must manage the stress in their lives before they can focus their energy on the lifestyle changes necessary to manage weight.

I disagree!

Managing stress is part of managing weight. Managing weight is part of managing stress. They are interlinked and must be addressed together.

The Six-Week Body-Signal Program

Week 1

Weight Focus: Your Hunger Signals; your Satisfaction Signals; chewing
Personal Focus: Scales; mirrors; eye contact
Nutrition Focus: Plotting the path to optimal health

Prepare for takeoff! You have a very busy and exciting week ahead of you.

Weight Focus

Your Hunger Signals. Since the first step toward controlling weight is knowing what a Hunger Signal *is* and where it's coming from, this week you're going to concentrate on learning to recognize a true Hunger Signal.

On the first day of the program, as soon as you awaken, check for a Hunger Signal. Don't automatically reach for your usual breakfast fare—you may or may not actually feel hunger! And you may feel confused. After all, you have years of ingrained habits to beat down.

Rapid refresher: Review "How to Know When You're Hungry" on page 146.

If you believe you're experiencing a Hunger Signal, go ahead and eat whatever you want. If you're not, wait until the next signal occurs, which may happen in the next ½ hour or at the end of the day. (You won't starve—don't worry.) Once you start to master this skill, you'll find that several times a day (usually about five or six) the body will call for fuel (food). The amounts vary each time.

The point for you to remember is this: No food should cross your lips unless there's a signal from your body. For now, your task is to get back in touch with this crucial signal and to make sure you always respond to it.

Bear in mind that you *must eat* when your body signals. Too many years of dieting have led many of you to believe you must "white-knuckle" it through your hunger. *Forget that practice!* Throughout the day, continue to eat whenever your hunger signals. Whether you fed yourself 3 minutes or 18 hours ago—if you feel that signal, eat. For now, it makes no difference if you overeat. (No, this is not permission to binge, but if you do—relax. Lighten up. It's okay.) The object is to begin accumulating experience with your Hunger Signals—to know them, to become intimate with them. Eventually, your body will regulate itself.

Again, it must be emphasized that you're a novice and your signals may be confusing. Depending on how many diets you've been on in your life, it could take weeks or even months to master this response. For this reason, your patience, perseverance, and practice is crucial. Without this skill, you have no chance of ever solving your weight problem! But don't worry. Each day of the program—and each week—you'll be moving closer to mastering your signals. Each day, you'll become more sensitized to them and more proficient at responding to them. Believe me—everyone learns this skill!

One more idea. Becoming intimate with your Hunger Signals will be much easier if you begin to suspend the dieter's judgment. You know what I mean. "I responded to my Hunger Signal—I was good," or "I overate or ate when I wasn't hungry—I was bad." These judgments must go! Your work isn't nullified by doing it "wrong."

You're learning a new skill. Go easy on yourself, and expect some confusion for a while.

Your Satisfaction Signals. This week, while your focus should be on your Hunger Signals, you also need to begin paying some attention to your Satisfaction (satiety) Signals. Your Hunger Signals are your first priority, because satiety is the *absence of hunger.* Before you can know when hunger is absent, you must know when it's present.

Rapid refresher: To help you focus in on your Satisfaction Signals, review "The Hunger Scale" on page 143.

If feasible, you may want to tape the exercises starting on page 143 and play them back to yourself with your eyes closed while you're in a relaxed setting.

Rapid refresher: Review "How to Know When You're Satisfied" on page 149.

Again, the Satisfaction Signal may confuse you. Since you're not accustomed to stopping the flow of the fork until your plate is clean, you probably don't know what a satiety response feels like.

The key to weight control is eating just the right amount of food to satisfy your body. Keep in mind that scientific studies have proven that the body knows just how to regulate how much it needs. When you respond to your body, you won't gain weight.

Go easy on yourself. It may take a while to fully recognize satisfaction.

Chewing. As bizarre as this topic sounds, the only way to fully master your Satisfaction Signals is to practice that most elusive of skills—*chewing!* Here's how.

- Starting today, after you feel a Hunger Signal and begin to eat, make your chewing *conscious.*
- Every time you eat, after each bite, put your fork, spoon, or sandwich down.
- Chew your food until it liquefies in your mouth before you go on to your next bite.

I fully believe that chewing is the most crucial skill an Overeater must master. The only way to know how much to eat is to eat slowly enough to be conscious of what your body is telling you.

This weekend, be on the lookout for unconscious and "polite" eating. Excess fat can easily be accumulated by bad timing. If much of what you eat ignores your Body Signals and much food is ingested unconsciously, you will gain excess weight.

Conscious eating means you're continuously asking the question: "Am I still hungry?" If the answer remains yes, keep on eating. When the answer becomes no, you've hit the point of satisfaction. It's time to stop.

When you stay conscious of what you are eating, you are able to gain control, and that control will allow you to eat just the right amount.

Personal Focus

Please note: For this section of the program, days 1, 3, and 5 have been designated for learning new behaviors or skills. Use the alternate days to reinforce your new practices. Since Saturdays and Sundays tend to be more relaxed for most people, to bolster your commitment, it's important to continue your work through the weekends.

Day 1: Scales. On the first day of the program, you'll want to be extremely clear as to the purpose of your actions. You'll want to prove to yourself that you:

- *Are* finally trashing the Diet Mentality
- *Do* accept yourself and are at peace with your acceptance
- *Are* entitled to fulfillment and high self-esteem
- *Will* effectively deal with others *without* feeling the need to apologize for yourself
- *Will* complete the tasks you set for yourself

Let's start.

Some months after graduating from my Lighten Up seminar, a woman named Melanie reported that she donned a dress she hadn't worn for a while and discovered it was now "hanging" on her. She was thrilled! "This had to mean I'd lost at least 20 pounds," she exclaimed. Immediately, she ran to the scale and gleefully weighed herself. "The scale registered a mere 2-pound loss," she said, and she instantly found herself in the throes of the Woman's Model. She was weight obsessed, had fallen back into the Diet Mentality, and was reexperiencing the female mandate for misery (see "The Woman's Model" on page 18).

Today, throw your scale in the trash!

No, that doesn't mean put it in the closet or basement (unless your spouse or some other family member insists on keeping it). Go for trashing the Diet Mentality 100 percent! Throw the scale away!

Day 3: Mirrors. Dolly weighs well above 200 pounds. A few weeks after graduating the seminar, she did something that, as she puts it, "blew me away!"

Like one of the Nancy/Carol scripts from chapter 5, after showering one evening, she walked into the bedroom where her husband was watching television. "That actress is one sexy woman!" he commented. Dolly didn't fold. Instead, she playfully sashayed his way and provocatively demanded, "Oh, yeah! And what about this sexy woman?!"

Today, look at your naked body in the mirror.

Start telling yourself the *truth* about your body (even if it doesn't *feel* like the truth—*yet*). Tell yourself out loud:

"I look beautiful!"

"Peter Paul Rubens really knew what sensuous was!"

"Someone would sure be lucky to cuddle with this body!"

"This body looks great moving, standing, sitting down!"

"This body is terrific!"

Or, add your own nurturing comments.

Continue to look in the mirror every day until *the truth feels like the truth!*

Day 5: Eye contact. The day after completing my seminar, Tania couldn't understand why those strangers at work were suddenly so friendly toward her. It started when she got out of her car in the company parking lot. Co-workers smiled and gave her friendly nods. When she entered the building, employees whom she'd never met during her five years at the company smiled, said "Good morning," and asked how she was doing. She was a bit bewildered by this outpouring of good will. Then the light bulb flashed on.

Tania realized that every day for the past five years, she had gotten out of her car with her eyes cast down to the ground, where they remained fixed until she reached her office. She never *saw* these people who had been seeing her for years.

Today, she was standing straight and making eye contact with everyone. Her new demeanor and awareness were drawing in their warm responses.

Today, start walking erect, with your head held high, and make eye contact with the people you encounter.

Continue making eye contact at work, at parties, in restaurants, at reunions, in aerobics class (but do remember to use discretion on the streets).

Nutrition Focus

Plotting the path to optimal health. You're about to read the most important nutritional directive you will ever learn in your entire life: *Change your nutritional lifestyle slowly—slowly—slowly.*

It took two years for me to overhaul mine. I suggest you only make one or two changes a month—give yourself the time you need to adjust. If quite suddenly you change your nutritional habits—clean out your shelves, then rush to the health food store and restock them with "healthy" foods—you'll experience emotional vertigo. *Don't rush your progress!* You don't want to find yourself spinning back into that desperate, out-of-control sensation.

For this reason, this week, I suggest you make no nutritional changes. Instead, each day list a few changes that you'd like to make in your nutritional repertoire a year or two down the road. Here are some start-up suggestions. Resolution—I will:

- Eat two-thirds to three-quarters of my daily food from high-fiber categories of fruits, vegetables, whole grains, and beans.
- Eat several servings of calcium-rich green vegetables (cruciferous vegetables) each day.
- Introduce a variety of fiber-rich beans into my diet.
- Experiment with all of the nutrient-dense whole grains and continue eating those that appeal to me every day.
- Eat two to three servings a week of fish rich in omega-3 fatty acids.
- Try eating free-range poultry and red meat from natural-grazing farm animals.
- Learn about snacks I can enjoy without fear and try limiting my treats to those foods.
- Experiment with fat and milk alternatives.

From this short list, you're sure to understand why I say, "Take it slowly!" If you think you'd like to make these nutritional changes in your life, then you'll want the tips and guidelines in the next few weeks of the program.

At the risk of being repetitious, let me say again that these tips and guidelines do not have to be implemented all at once—all within six weeks. They are designed to let you pick and choose at your own comfortable pace.

Week 2

Weight Focus: The Body-Signal eating guidelines; handling sugar cravings
Personal Focus: Clothes that don't fit; asking for and getting what you want; using the Three R's
Nutrition Focus: Enjoying taboos: snacks

Week 1 review: How regularly did you:

- Locate your Hunger Signals?
- Respond to your Satisfaction Signals?
- Chew your food thoroughly?

Look at your answers without judgment and see if you can do better this week.

Weight Focus

The Body-Signal eating guidelines. The backbone of mastering your Satisfaction Signals is the Body-Signal eating guidelines. If you consistently follow them, you'll have to remain focused on your body's hunger/satisfaction needs.

If you do nothing else, follow the Body-Signal eating guidelines!

Rapid refresher: Right now, flip back and review "Be Deliberately Conscious of Food" and "The Body-Signal Eating Guidelines," on page 153.

Handling sugar cravings. If you experience sugar cravings or a "sweet tooth," deciding to reduce or eliminate refined sugar is easier said than done. You must learn how to manage that craving.

Although we eat food to satisfy hunger, when it comes to sweets, that's often not the case. Sweets satisfy a different need—it may be taste, titillation, you name it. But no matter what you call it, for those of us with a sweet tooth, sweets are a major pleasure.

For some of you, the desire to pleasure yourself with sweets is a sometime thing. For others, it's a need akin to addiction.

Your total goal here is to develop a take-it-or-leave-it attitude toward sugary foods. That way, when you decide to eat it, you'll be in control, you'll enjoy it, you'll feel no guilt, and you'll eat the right amount to pleasure yourself appropriately. Here's the easiest way to control the craving.

For at least three days, include a lot of high-fiber foods in your repertoire. These foods include legumes, whole grains, and dark green vegetables. Bear in mind that during this week, *there's no way you could eat too much brown rice or broccoli!* And for this three-day period *only,* eat *no* fruit or yeast-containing products (read labels).

By following this plan, many Lighten Up seminar graduates have reported that their sugar cravings disappeared.

In case you have difficulty the first day, keep a couple of cooked chicken legs in the refrigerator. When you crave sugar, munching on a chicken leg will help you get over the craving.

Please note: If you give this plan a try and still feel you must have sugar, go ahead and have some. Relax about it and start over the next day.

In the future, you'll find that when you make a choice to eat sugar, you can cut the cravings by immediately returning to this process. If you've been sugar-free for some time, you should lose your craving in one day.

Give these instructions a try and see if you can totally eliminate refined sugar from your diet for five days (without feeling as if you were abusing yourself on a sugar-deprivation diet.)

Personal Focus

Day 1: Clothes that don't fit. Are you willing to do 100 percent of what it takes? When seminar participants hear what their next task is, invariably a chorus of groans and excuses rises in the room.

Being powerful means being who you are *today*—not holding yourself in reserve until you become the fantasy you of tomorrow.

Today, only one size of clothes fits you. Any clothes of any other size belong to someone else with someone else's body. If you accept yourself as you are today, these clothes have no business being in your closet.

Today, throw away, give away, or swap any clothes you own that don't fit you!

If you only want to be a 95 percenter—and why would you?—then at least pack them in a trunk and store them in the attic.

Day 3: Asking for and getting what you want. When Marla was handed a new project by her boss, she quickly realized she needed some help. She approached her boss and said, "Jan, if I'm going to do this job right, I need an assistant to manage the legwork."

Her boss replied: "Marla, you'll have to do the best you can on your own."

Marla came to a seminar session still frustrated by her boss's response. During the weekend, she learned what I like to call the Three R's of Asking—Recognition, Requirement, Request.

After the seminar, she returned to her boss and said, "Jan, I know you're under a lot of pressure to hold expenses down and avoid unnecessary hiring, and I'm on your side on those points. If I'm going to do this job right, I need an assistant to manage the legwork. Will you give me permission to hire an assistant?"

This time her approach was a completely different story. The first time around, Marla only stated her requirement. There was no way her boss could have sensed that Marla recognized any other corporate concerns or that she even gave a hoot. Nor did Marla ask for what she wanted. She never said, "Can I have an assistant?" As a result, she never received a yes or no answer.

The Three R's greatly increase your chances of getting what you want. (By the way, the third R is *request*—not *demand*. Your tone must make it clear that you are requesting a yes, not demanding it.)

Today, use the Three R's and ask someone for something you want.

Day 5: Using the Three R's. The difference between successful people and those who are not boils down to this: Successful people have a greater capacity to endure frustration and rejection.

Today, continue using the Three R's to ask for what you want.

Here are some suggestions.

- Ask your boss for a raise or promotion.
- If you're the family cook, ask your mate to take you out to eat at a restaurant once for every five dinners you cook.
- Create a fantasy in which you're having a wonderful sexual experience. Make it specific. Now ask your mate to live out the fantasy with you.
- Tell your mate that you'd like to satisfy him sexually. Ask what you can do to make this happen.
- You've been demanding that your child perform a certain task. Now, using the Three R's, *ask* him or her to take care of it.

The more you ask for what you want, the more you may hear no. But of course, the more you ask, the more you also invite a series of yes answers.

Nutrition Focus

Enjoying taboos: snacks. You're now about to read the second most important nutritional fact you will ever learn in your entire life: *There's nothing edible on this planet that you can't eat!* (Barring individual food sensitivities, of course.)

Changing your nutrition intake to predominantly high-fiber foods doesn't constitute a new "diet." It's now time to stop thinking in terms of good foods versus taboo foods. Instead, how about putting foods into one of the following three categories.

1. Foods you consider to be healthy. These foods can be eaten in unlimited quantities based on the demands of your Body Signals.
2. Foods that don't meet your standard of healthy nutrition. These are

foods you can comfortably do without—and still not feel deprived (for me, two examples are margarine and pork).
3. Foods that don't meet your standard of healthy nutrition but that you *cannot* comfortably do without (my two examples are ice cream and bagels made with enriched flour).

Think of it this way. You're going to choose to eat two-thirds to three-quarters of your food from the healthy, high-fiber group. For the greater proportion of the remaining one-third to one-quarter of your diet, you're going to choose healthy, low-fiber foods (nuts, seeds, vegetable oils, dairy products, fish, poultry, meat). The small percentage that's left will accommodate the so-called unhealthy foods.

This means that because your diet will now overwhelmingly consist of healthy foods, you will have created a safety net that will allow you to enjoy foods in your third category without guilt.

You'll be able to eat and *enjoy* these foods without feeling deprived *and* without worrying that you're overindulging yourself.

Think of the foods you habitually eat and assign them to one of the three categories.

Week 3

Weight Focus: Eating what your body wants
Personal Focus: New responses to old comments; new clothes; medical care
Nutrition Focus: Food tips for the working person

Weeks 1 and 2 review: How regularly did you:

• Locate your Hunger Signals?
• Respond to your Satisfaction Signals?
• Chew your food thoroughly?
• Eat sugar?

Look at your answers without judgment and see if you can do better this week.

Weight Focus

Eating what your body wants. If you don't eat what you (and your body) want, you won't feel satisfied. If you don't feel satisfied, you'll overeat to compensate for your unfulfilled food needs and ignore your Body Signals.

For this reason, you need to practice eating what you truly want.

Rapid refresher: Review "How to Eat What You Really Want" on page 150 and "Food Minefields" on page 152.

Obviously, you don't always have a choice in the matter. If you're a guest at someone's home (or even when you're in your own home), you may be served a limited number of items. In general, however, if you choose the foods you really want and eat just the right amount to satisfy yourself, you'll enjoy food without gaining weight.

There is one catch to all this—and it's a big one. What happens when your body seems to crave sweets? (Don't worry. We'll cover this problem in week 4.)

Go through the "How to Eat What You Really Want" checklist on page 150 and identify what your body is asking for. If possible, avoid eating any food that doesn't flash through your mind before you see it.

Personal Focus

Day 1: New responses to old comments. Earlier in this book, you read about the seminar graduate who sent us a letter telling about her low self-esteem, which had previously permitted people to "walk all over her." If you recall, she reported that after the seminar, her situation had totally changed. As she put it, "Now that I'm feeling so feisty again, I actually *want* people to mess with me."

Review in your mind the comments and criticisms you've been subjected to from well-meaning and not-so-well-meaning people. Since you've now replaced your "walking apology" attitude with a feeling of dignity and an attitude of self-respect, imagine what you'd do if one of those situations came up now.

Today, create new responses to inappropriate comments about your body and eating behaviors.

Here are a few suggestions.

"Thank you. I agree that I look great since I lost this weight, but I also thought I looked great before I lost it—didn't you?"

"What I eat is not up for discussion!"

"I really can't add anything to this discussion because I don't diet."

"Is that all you can think of to say to me?"

"You must be blind! This body is absolutely fine the way it is!"

Day 3: New clothes. At last! Designers have finally gotten wise to the fact that the average woman is size 14 to 16. There are more beautiful, chic clothes in great fabrics for larger-size women than ever before in the fashion industry.

If you were to dress to *flaunt* your beauty (instead of hiding your defects), what colors would you wear? What fabrics would you choose? What styles?

Today, take yourself out clothes shopping. Confine your purchases to items that make you feel great. Buy something in a different color, fabric, or style.

Day 5: Medical care. Take care of your body—treat it the way you would treat your child. You should visit your internist for a checkup every two years and your gynecologist every year. Depending on your age group, find out how frequently you should have a mammogram performed. Ask questions about yourself. Don't put these appointments off.

Today, call and make appointments if you are overdue for a checkup.

A reminder: If the doctor insists on weighing you, step on the scale backward and tell the doctor you're not interested in knowing the number.

Nutrition Focus

Food tips for the working person. Even with an ever-busy schedule, you don't have to sacrifice healthy eating. Your snacks, lunches, and dinners can still consist of low-fat, high-fiber, vitamin-rich foods.

For midmorning/midafternoon snacks:

- Take a container of plain, low-fat yogurt mixed with high-fiber cereal, raisins, cinnamon, and lemon or almond extract to your office with you. Mix it the night before.
- Leave a package of rice cakes, almond butter, and a plastic knife in your desk drawer. When you're hungry, just reach in and fix a quick snack.
- On the days when the vending machine is your only snack recourse, avoid the candy bars—select raisins or popcorn.

For brown-bag lunches:

- Make yourself a sandwich. Use multigrain, rye, or whole wheat bread with chicken, turkey, or tuna as a filler.
- Pack some RyKrisp or stone-ground wafers in your bag or briefcase along with raw carrots, celery, and zucchini sticks. Don't forget some fresh fruit.

When eating lunch out:

- Try a restaurant or deli with a salad bar. Choose dark salad greens, broccoli, carrots, beets, garbanzo beans, or a little chicken salad.
- Order a chicken or turkey sandwich and a cup of vegetable or bean soup.

- At a Chinese restaurant, order brown rice and a stir-fried dish with lots of vegetables.
- If you're going for fast food, order a baked potato and top it with vegetables, yogurt, or chili.

For dinner:

- On your days off, cook in quantity and freeze pots of soup, chili, or whole wheat, spinach, or artichoke pasta in individual containers. If you feel like baking, double all your recipes for whole-grain muffins and breads and freeze individual portions.
- If you don't have a microwave, you might want to consider investing in one. Microwave your food and your Hunger Signals won't have to wait.

Week 4

Weight Focus: Reading the labels; getting around in the health food stores; more help handling sugar cravings
Personal Focus: Turning "failure" into feedback; bathing suits; procrastination
Nutrition Focus: Snacks: tips for Mom and Dad

Weeks 1, 2, and 3 review: How regularly did you:

- Locate your Hunger Signals?
- Respond to your Satisfaction Signals?
- Chew your food thoroughly?
- Eat sugar?
- Eat what your body really wanted?

Look at your answers without judgment and see if you can do better this week.

Weight Focus

Reading the labels. Ultimately, the foundation of managing weight requires two steps: responding to your Hunger/Satisfaction Signals and controlling (not necessarily eliminating) sugar and excess fat.

You probably don't yet comprehend just how much sugar you do eat. Maybe you're one of those people who use that oft-repeated refrain, "I only take a couple of teaspoons in my coffee." But according to the studies, you could be eating from 60 to 120 pounds of sugar a year— 20 percent of your entire food intake!

So where is it hidden? You need to know. You can't cut down on sugar if you don't know where it is! To find the enemy—*read labels!*

When you check out the labels on cans, jars, boxes, and packages in the supermarket, you notice something very odd. Items in aisles 1, 2, 3, and 4 all contain many of the same ingredients—sugars, fatty hydrogenated oils, artificial flavors, and salt. Without these ingredients, a huge percentage of the nonmeat and nonproduce foods would disappear from the shelves—they'd simply be tasteless.

The ingredients in any packaged food are listed on the label in order of highest to lowest quantity. Once you start reading labels, you might be shocked to discover the number one ingredient isn't always what you think you're buying! For instance, the number one ingredient in many breakfast cereals isn't cereal—it's sugar!

Consumers are frequently misled about the amounts of sweeteners in products. When you add up all the different forms of sugar, you'll find that some products are 95 percent sweetener.

All of the following items are actually sugar. *Learn these aliases:* sucrose, dextrose, fructose, maltose, high-fructose corn syrup, corn syrup, corn sweetener, honey, molasses, maple syrup, invert syrup, brown sugar, turbinado sugar, raw sugar.

Okay. Let's move on to breads, pastas, more cereals, baked goods, and "white" sauces. You now know that refined wheat flour, or white flour, appears to promote weight gain. If this substance has been added to a product, it can be identified by the word "enriched."

You've also learned about the danger of fats. Hydrogenation is a man-made process in which hydrogen is added to polyunsaturated oils, turning them into saturated oils. There is good experimental evidence demonstrating that these oils can be toxic and promote cancer and heart disease. For this reason, margarine is on the list of foods I never eat.

When you begin to read the labels on your favorite products, you'll see that many are made with the most highly saturated oils. Coconut oil is included—it's more saturated than beef tallow—as well as palm oil, cottonseed oil, and partially hydrogenated soybean oil.

Now let's deal with salt. Remember that processed foods may be the highest source of salt in the American diet!

And a word about artificial colors and flavors. These two additives are generally regarded as safe. Still, their presence on a label does raise the question about the quality of the food and its taste—why, you wonder, is it necessary to add them?

You should definitely stay alert to the addition of all artificial sweeteners.

It's no secret that you'll find artificial sweeteners in colas—but they're not the only item on the cola label that should alert you. When you read cola labels, you'll often find phosphoric acid, a substance that may lead to osteoporosis (softening of the bones).

To summarize, the categories to make note of are sweeteners, artificial sweeteners, enriched flour, hydrogenated oils, saturated oils, artificial colors and flavors, and phosphoric acid.

One more note about labels. Check on how many grams of fat are in the product. If this number is greater than 15 percent of the total, you may want to shove the item back on the shelf. (Remember, fat has twice as many calories as protein and carbohydrate, so an item that is 15 percent fat actually supplies 30 percent of the calories as fat.) Since labeling is not required to tell you how many calories come from fat, this is probably the best quick way to figure whether the item contains too much fat.

On the front page of the *New York Times* (March 8, 1990), Secretary of Health and Human Services Louis W. Sullivan, M.D., was quoted as saying: "The grocery store has become a Tower of Babel, and consumers need to be linguists, scientists, and mind readers to understand the many labels they see. Vital information is missing, and frankly, some unfounded health claims are being made."

Dr. Sullivan has outlined what he calls "a comprehensive reform of the nation's food labeling." But until his plan goes into effect, you'll have to be your own "fat calculator."

When you go food shopping, be sure to read all labels. (To get a jump-start, you may want to read labeled items currently sitting on your shelves at home.)

Getting around in the health food stores. Do you eat cereal? Bread? Cake? Pie? Cookies? Pasta? Items like these in supermarkets are almost always made with "enriched" white flour. Health food stores, however, frequently stock products made with whole grains. Pasta is a good example. In supermarkets, it's usually "enriched." Not so in health food stores. You can find whole wheat pasta, spinach pasta, artichoke pasta, and sometimes a few other tasty choices.

When you shop in health food stores, you'll find that many of your favorite products are sweetened with barley malt, rice syrup, date juice, or natural fruit juice—not fructose. These natural sweeteners have three major advantages: they're usually found in vitamin-rich, high-fiber foods; there's no evidence to suggest that they cause the problems that refined sugars do; and they taste delicious, without being *too* sweet.

You might want to note that a lot of foods in health food stores are sweetened with honey or molasses. Be aware that these two items are no better for you than refined sugar.

Today's health food store is really nothing more than yesterday's local food market. It offers foods (unrefined grains and free-range poultry, for example) that until recently were missing from supermarket shelves. However, major supermarket chains have become aware of a shifting consumer demand for better nutrition, and now they, too, are stocking many of the same items.

Health food stores are certainly no panacea for the ills of the marketplace. In many, the prices are greatly inflated. They do, however, offer alternatives to supermarket foods. Consider these stores specialty shops—places where you can buy a variety of whole-grain products, beans, naturally sweetened desserts and snacks, and free-range poultry. A lot of these foods (particularly the poultry) taste much better—they're more flavorful.

If you're not used to health food shopping, make your initial forays once-a-month trips. Pick busy health food stores where the turnover is fast and the food is most likely to be fresh.

More help handling sugar cravings. The best way to remain sugar-free is to fill your refrigerator and cupboards with foods sweetened with barley malt, natural fruit juice, and other natural sweeteners such as those mentioned above.

Take a trip to the health food store. Read the labels. Stock up on the foods you enjoy. For example, if you like cookies, buy some that are sweetened with fruit juice. Just knowing these foods are handy and available will help you avoid the panic of feeling "goodie" deprived.

Please note: You may have to experiment with different varieties before finding the most appealing foods for your palate. Give yourself time. Developing a taste for new foods may take a while. Eventually, however, many people do find they can't go back to their old favorites— they say the old refined-sugar products they used to love now taste "sickeningly" sweet.

Personal Focus

Day 1: Turning "failure" into feedback. No one's perfect! Or more accurately—no one does everything perfectly right.

There is no task for today—but there is something important to think about.

There's a good probability that as you finish the third week of the program, you've already binged or overeaten. If you haven't, you will in the weeks ahead.

How will you respond to that binge? With Mental Hara-Kiri? Negative judgments?

Don't do it! Remember: Binges are an "old" way of taking care of yourself. You may still need to "use" binges from time to time. *That's fine.* You're a beginner.

If you regard a binge as a failure, let's change it—let's turn that "failure" into feedback. From now on, after a binge, think about what preceded it. Ask yourself, "What was I taking care of? Is there a lesson to be learned?" For example:

• Did I feel deprived?
• Was I afraid I'd feel deprived?
• Did something frighten me?
• Was I experiencing an emotion that was difficult for me to handle?

Whatever it was, just make sure it's identified and that you understand the binge was taking care of it.

Remind yourself that you didn't fail by bingeing. And remember that if you take the time to reflect, the episode will provide you with valuable feedback. In the future, when that same feeling emerges, what alternative response will you choose? An attitude of failure perpetuates binges. Feedback permits you to slowly but surely assuage the need to binge.

Day 3: Bathing suits. If the season is right, wear a bathing suit in public. If not, model it for your mirror.

Today, wear a bathing suit! Enjoy the experience!

If the Internal Saboteur has something to say about it, create and recite new lyrics. Some suggestions:

"What a beautiful woman!"
"I look great!"
"That's a helluva sexy body!"

Day 5: Procrastination. What have you been putting off? Your taxes? Balancing your checkbook? Making those phone calls? Cleaning the _____?

It's time to motivate yourself to *just do it!*

Rapid refresher: Review the motivation techniques in chapter 5. Use the techniques.

Today, complete the task you've been putting off!

Nutrition Focus

Snacks: tips for Mom and Dad. How do you beat down those television commercials screaming out inducements for sugary snacks and junk food? As a parent who's becoming more health conscious, you're going to want to set some good examples for the kids. Teaching your children to eat well means practicing what you preach.

Here are some tips for making good nutrition a family affair.

• Keep foods such as fresh fruits, whole-grain muffins, and sliced raw vegetables handy.

- For soft drinks, try club soda mixed with unsweetened fruit juices. If you like, you can add some cubed fruit to the drink.
- Grapes are a winning item with kids. Put some seedless grapes in small paper cups, then fill the cups with their favorite fruit juice. Partially freeze, then insert sticks in the center and freeze until firm.
- Offer them a cantaloupe shake: Place ½ cup chilled, unsweetened pineapple juice and 2 cups chilled, cubed cantaloupe chunks in your blender. It's delicious and looks great!

Week 5

Weight Focus: Handling "fattening" foods
Personal Focus: Programming for success
Nutrition Focus: Navigating a restaurant menu

Weeks 1, 2, 3, and 4 review: How regularly did you:

- Locate your Hunger Signals?
- Respond to your Satisfaction Signals?
- Chew your food thoroughly?
- Eat sugar?
- Eat what your body really wanted?
- Read labels?
- Eat naturally sweetened foods?

Look at your answers without judgment and see if you can do better this week.

Weight Focus

Handling "fattening" foods. Sugar. Fat. Alcohol. Artificial sweeteners. "Enriched" white flour. Fried foods.

These are the weight-gain culprits.

It's time for you to decide what you're going to do about them. Keep in mind there is no such thing as a taboo food. But these substances appear to cause weight problems when eaten in excessive quantities by susceptible individuals. What quantities do you feel are appropriate for you?

Spend this week thinking about the answer to that question. Take into consideration health, weight, and your feelings (particularly feelings of deprivation). Then fill in the blanks on the following "fattening" foods commitment list. Promise—I will:

- Consume sugary foods a maximum of _____ times a week.
- Eat a maximum of _____ percent of my diet as fat.

- Drink a maximum of _____ alcoholic beverages a month.
- Eat fried foods a maximum of _____ times a month.
- Drink a maximum of _____ colas a month.
- Eat artificially sweetened foods a maximum of _____ times a month.
- Eat "enriched" foods a maximum of _____ times a month.

Now it's time to establish your commitment to respond to your Body Signals. (Remember—you can change these numbers as you go along.) Just fill in the blanks in the following Body-Signal commitment list. Promise—I will:

- Attempt to locate my Hunger Signal _____ times a day, _____ days a week.
- Eat in response to my Hunger Signals _____ percent of the time.
- Respond to my Satisfaction Signals _____ percent of the time.
- Adhere to the Body-Signal eating guidelines for _____ percent of my meals.
- Post the Body-Signal eating guidelines (page 153) on the refrigerator (optional).
- Go through my checklist for what I really want to eat (page 151) _____ times a week.

Personal Focus

After four weeks on the program, no doubt you have the day-to-day routine pretty well in hand. It's time for you to graduate from daily directives to a broader view. With that in mind, for each of these last two weeks, I'll focus on one important principle and/or valuable technique that will smooth your path to Instinctive Eater status.

Programming for success. Last week you started yourself on a task-completion "roll." This week, keep going. Identify a long-term project you wish to complete. For example:

- Respond to Body Signals.
- Schedule an exercise program.
- Create a business plan.
- Develop a project or plan at work.

Rapid refresher: Review "Programming Yourself to Succeed: The Time Machine" on page 115.

Today, place yourself 6 to 12 months into the future and describe how you overcame the obstacles necessary to complete the project. Now start.

Nutrition Focus

Navigating a restaurant menu. Eating out doesn't have to be an out-of-control experience. In fact, when it's done right, it can be a healthy, nutritious, and extremely tasty experience.

Here are five basic suggestions.

1. Think about what you would like to eat *before* looking at the restaurant menu.
2. Scan the menu for items that will fill that bill and meet your nutritional standards. The approach should be moderation—not deprivation!
3. Your meal doesn't have to be selected from the listed entrées. You may want to combine a few appetizers or side dishes to form your meal.
4. Feel free to take charge of your ordering. If you're avoiding sugar, salt, and margarine, don't hesitate to ask the server if these are used in preparing foods. If any of these ingredients are part of sauces, for example, ask that the sauce be omitted or served on the side. That way you can control the amount you eat.
5. Your best bets in nonethnic restaurants are light soups, salads, vegetables, beans, deep-sea fish, and poultry—baked, broiled, roasted, steamed, poached, or stir-fried.

If you have occasion to dine at ethnic restaurants, you may need additional guidance. Here are some special tips for a few of my favorite cuisines.

Chinese. Your best bets are steamed, poached, or stir-fried dishes. Try to avoid deep-fried foods (wontons, egg rolls, shrimp toast) as well as spareribs.

Italian. Again, look for items that are steamed or poached, and sauces such as marinara, marsala, or cacciatore. Try to avoid sausage and breaded or fried foods.

Greek. If you're going for kabobs, avoid the beef and ask for the chicken. If you seldom eat meat, take this opportunity to indulge yourself by ordering the delicious lamb!

Indian. Your best bet here is anything tandoori, which means the chicken or shrimp is slow-cooked with yogurt. You can also find a good variety of vegetable dishes. My favorite is *aloo, mutter-gobi* (a vegetable combo).

Japanese. Try to avoid anything tempura—deep-fried shrimp or vegetables. And although raw fish served Japanese-style is delicious, there is some danger of contracting hepatitis from it, so avoid it for your own safety.

Week 6

Weight Focus: Exercise
Personal Focus: Forgiveness
Nutrition Focus: Preparing to fly on your own!

Weeks 1, 2, 3, 4, and 5 review: How regularly did you:

- Locate your Hunger Signals?
- Respond to your Satisfaction Signals?
- Chew your food thoroughly?
- Eat sugar?
- Eat what your body really wanted?
- Read labels?
- Eat naturally sweetened foods?
- Stick to your "fattening" foods commitments?

Look at your answers without judgment and see if you can do better this week.

Weight Focus

Exercise. I've already discussed the pros and cons of exercise for weight control in chapter 10 (see the exercise and weight section on page 172 and "Major Benefits of Exercise" on page 174). Now I'll address some of the specifics.

What type of exercise should you be doing? You must do aerobic exercise. If you're not sure what aerobic exercise actually means, here's a practical definition: continuous exercise in which you work up a sweat.

Strengthening exercises, such as weight training and Nautilus, do build strength, but they don't provide the benefits I listed. Flexibility exercises, such as yoga or stretching, will limber you up, but they don't provide the other overall improvements in fitness either. Nearly all sports are ineffective or inefficient for improving fitness.

Aerobic exercises include cross-country skiing and simulators, rowing machines, and swimming—they're good because they work the upper and lower body. But also think about running, jogging, race walking, rapid bicycling, stationary bicycling at a rapid pace or against resistance equivalent to a slight uphill grade, calisthenics, aerobic dancing, video aerobic workouts, aerobics classes, and the treadmills and Stairmaster equipment featured at many gyms.

How many days should you be exercising? Compared to *no* exercise, one or two days a week of aerobic exercise provides only slight, if any, improvement in fitness. But three days will result in a big leap in fitness levels. Four days will provide another big jump—though not as great as the leap from two to three days.

At five, six, and seven days a week, fitness levels do increase, but the returns diminish significantly in terms of the effort invested.

If you want to do the minimum amount of exercise to become fit and stay fit, do the exercise three times a week. If you want to receive the optimal return on your exercise investment, do it four times a week. (This is how often I include aerobics in my regimen.)

To train for an amateur athletic event, do aerobic exercise five times a week. In general, if you're doing heavy aerobic training, it's wise to rest two days a week. If you're exercising five or more days a week now, that means either that you know what you're doing and don't need my advice on how to start an exercise program, or you have some form of exercise bulimia. (This is a compulsive need to overexercise born from the mistaken notion that the more you exercise, the more calories you'll burn off.) If you follow the Body-Signal Program, you will be able to cut exercise time without gaining weight or sacrificing fitness.

How long should an exercise session last? The minimum exercise session should be 25 to 35 minutes, and your heart should be beating at its aerobic "training" rate (see page 248) for at least 12 minutes. Since it takes 5 to 10 minutes to warm up and 10 minutes to cool down (to prevent blood from "pooling" in the muscles), 25 to 35 minutes is necessary to achieve the 12 minutes at the training rate.

I don't recommend the minimum. I recommend a duration of exercise that will ensure 20 "aerobic" minutes—a good level to maintain and improve fitness for noncompeting individuals.

The longer you exercise, the more fit you'll become. Should you increase your time beyond a 35-minute session? That's up to you to determine.

How do you get started if you're unaccustomed to exercise? If you are not used to exercise, try a program of minutes on/minutes off. Start by exercising for 2 minutes and walking (or even resting) for 2 minutes, for a total of 16 minutes (8 minutes of actual exercising). Start increasing the total number of minutes. Also, you may want to shift the number of minutes on and off (3 on/2 off, 4 on/2 off, 3 on/1 off, 4 on/1 off, 5 on/2 off, 5 on/1 off, and so on). Base your shifts on what you can tolerate.

When you can exercise for 15 minutes, stop the rest periods. Begin to add 1 or 2 minutes every two weeks until you build up to 35 minutes.

How do you avoid overexercising? If you're not currently exercising, start your exercise program at a reasonable pace. This means that 5 to 10 minutes after completing your exercise session, your breathing should be back to normal and you should feel much the way you did before the session started.

The exercise should feel like work; you should be slightly winded but not gasping. Your heart should be fast but not racing or thumping in your chest; you should feel mild discomfort but not fatigue or pain. (By the way, if you can talk as you exercise, you're not exercising too hard. And if you can sing, you aren't exercising hard enough.)

If you experience light-headedness, dizziness, near-fainting, or chest pain, stop immediately! Don't resume exercise until after you've consulted your physician about it.

After meals, wait at least 30 minutes to an hour before exercising. After finishing your exercise session, cool down by walking or stretching for 10 to 15 minutes. Except to stretch, never lie down or sit immediately after exercising. If you do some stretching, it should always be done after exercise, not before. This will prevent muscle pulls.

How do you prevent underexercising? There is a formula for determining your training heart rate (pulse): 220 minus your age times .75. Here are some examples.

At 20 years old: $220 - 20 = 200 \times .75 = 150$

At 40 years old: $220 - 40 = 180 \times .75 = 135$

Personally, I find that doing arithmetic and feeling for pulse rates while I exercise is a pain. I prefer to tune in to the wisdom of my Body Signals—to stay in touch with my body.

If my exercise is continuous (as it must be to be aerobic—except for beginners), and if I'm sweating enough to get my shirt wet—even in cold weather—then I know I'm getting a good workout. If my heart is beating hard but not thumping out of my chest, if my breathing is fast but even, and if my body is working hard and tiring but not exhausting itself, then I know I'm getting a good workout.

Do remember that routine activities—walking a lot and even climbing stairs throughout the day—can't be considered aerobic exercise. You must do formal exercise to reap the benefits. Don't be fooled by those who tell you that all you need to do is walk. If you're going to use walking as your form of exercise, you must do it briskly, aerobically, using appropriately supportive walking shoes, and perhaps even learn proper form.

Remember, to maintain good fitness and to reap the benefits of aerobic exercise, work up to 35 minutes, three or four times a week.

Choose the form(s) of aerobic exercise you intend to do. Schedule the minutes and days you will do this exercise. Start your exercise program.

Personal Focus

Forgiveness. You will end the final week of the Body-Signal Program by ridding yourself of the last burden dragging you down. You've done this program because you wanted to move on with your life free of the obsessions and the self-imposed anchors that keep you mired in unwanted feelings and behaviors. Now you're going to take the last step—the step that will free you to move on and fulfill your ambitions as a free, unfettered individual. Your final task:

Today, forgive everyone you have not yet forgiven—including yourself.
Don't forgive because it's moral.
And don't do it because it's ethical.
Forgive these people because it's practical—and it's essential for *your* well-being.
I'm not saying condone. I'm not saying suppress anger. I'm not saying call them up and confront them!
Forgiveness is not about *them*—it's about *you*!
The person who's suffering from nonforgiveness is *you*. The abusive father, the betraying ex-spouse, the neglectful mother—they're all inessential to you in the present—whether he or she is suffering or not.
Nonforgiveness is active and eroding. Obsessing, fantasizing revenge, constructing bad outcomes about the con artist who stole your life savings, is wasting your precious, valuable energy. What that person is doing now is irrelevant. What you're allowing him or her to do to you is critical. You've made this person an important part of your life. How ironic. You've ended up insisting that the person toward whom you have the least goodwill will remain a meaningful player in your life.
When you choose *non*forgiveness, you're making a declaration: "I choose to continue to be your victim; I choose to relate to you as though you are big and powerful and I am small and weak; I choose to use nonforgiveness as the defense against your power over me."
On the other hand, when you choose forgiveness, you're declaring: "It's over! I detach from you and your power over me. I am nobody's victim. I am big enough and powerful enough to forgive and to get on with my life without you to push up against. If you are still part of my life, I'm no longer willing to hand over my power to you.
"I don't need nonforgiveness or even anger to prevent you from

hurting me or my loved ones. I am powerful enough to forgive you and still be protected from you."

When we go through this particular event during the seminars, there are a lot of tight muscles, clenched jaws, and flowing tears—believe it.

Forgiveness *is* a major step—and often a difficult one. It's not a process. It's simply a sincere declaration, silently or verbally uttered: "I forgive you."

It's the difference between emotional and mental bondage and freedom.

To move on with your life fully, *you must forgive.* It makes no difference how much you fight it, refuse it, resist it, or justify your stance. The bottom line is this: If you don't forgive, *you're the only one who loses!*

When you forgive, you'll experience an incredible release, a profound relief, a deep feeling that you are truly in control of your life, and a certainty that the need for struggle is over.

Nutrition Focus

Preparing to fly on your own! You don't have to take a Magical Mystery Tour to arrive at a nutritious lifestyle!

In week 2, you began to think nutritiously by planning a diet of (1) predominantly high-fiber foods, (2) a variety of low-fiber foods, and (3) a dash of processed low-vitamin/low-mineral/high-fat/high-calorie foods, as they say, "just for the taste of it."

Good nutrition consists of give and take: Take away a lot of 3 foods (as you've already begun to do); add a variety of 1 and 2 foods. This means that over the coming years, you have the pleasurable task of adding delicious new foods to your repertoire.

While you're scanning the new possibilities for your palate, you might want to refer to the food lists in chapter 12. For instance:

Deep-sea fish. Eating two or three servings a week, even as little as 8 ounces a week, is a tasty, healthy idea. Bake, broil, poach, steam, microwave, or pan-fry using a quality vegetable oil such as olive, sesame, sunflower, or safflower.

Don't forget canned sardines, salmon, and tuna (packed in water).

Be creative with your seasonings. Consider basil, chives, dill, garlic, ginger, leeks, sweet onions, oregano, mustard sauce, saffron, scallions, and tomatoes.

Meat. Select low-fat cuts. For maximum tenderness, these lean cuts need slow, moist cooking. Marinate overnight for better flavor. Roast, braise, stew, or broil.

In my home, we eat meat loaf made with skinned, ground chicken and turkey. Light meat is half as fat as dark meat. You can also lower fat content by adding fillers such as soybean protein, bran, oatmeal, or wheat germ.

Instead of supermarket meat from animals raised in factories (feedlots) and treated with hormones, antibiotics, and other chemicals, try serving meat and poultry from animals raised naturally on farms. (I find the difference in flavor extraordinary.)

Keep your meat intake to 4-ounce servings. Trim all fat before cooking. After cooking, if you chill the dish, the excess fat from broths and stews will coagulate and rise to the surface, making it easy to skim off. Substitute herbs and spices for fat-filled gravies and sauces.

Don't forget variety! Try poultry, lamb, veal, even rabbit and venison. But go easy on pork and ham, and avoid packaged lunch meats.

Cheese. Stick with hard cheeses. Soft cheeses—Brie and Port Salut, for example—are generally rich in milk fat. Processed cheese, such as American and cream cheese, may contain undesirable ingredients.

Beans and legumes. Start planning meals around the wide variety of legumes available to you. With the exception of lentils and split peas, dried beans should be presoaked. First wash the beans, then place them in 4 parts water to 1 part beans and soak overnight in a covered pan. (To speed things up, bring the beans and water to a boil and cook for 2 minutes, then cover, remove from heat, and let stand for an hour.) Soaking helps reduce the formation of objectionable gas in beans.

To cook, drain and rinse the beans, then add fresh water to a level 2 inches above the beans and bring to a boil. Reduce heat, cover, and simmer slowly until tender. (Approximate cooking times: lentils–½ to 1 hour; lima beans–½ to 1½ hours; red or kidney beans–1½ to 2 hours; navy beans–1½ to 2 hours; pinto beans–2 to 2½ hours; garbanzos beans and soybeans–2 to 3 hours.) You can also pressure-cook beans, except limas. If you use canned beans, rinse them first to remove salt.

To save time, cook large amounts of beans and refrigerate for up to four days, or freeze for up to six months.

Legumes and grains are a tasty and nutritious combination. Try beans and whole wheat pasta, chili with cornbread, lentils and brown rice.

Winter greens. These nutrient-rich foods should be bought crisp and green, with no signs of wilting. They can be refrigerated, unwashed, for up to a week by wrapping them lightly in dampened paper towels and placing them inside a plastic bag that's been perforated to allow air to enter.

Four to 8 minutes of steaming produces tender, firm greens. To get around the bitter aftertaste of some winter greens, try microwaving or boiling them, uncovered, for 10 minutes. Then chop them up and sauté in olive oil and garlic with a dash of nutmeg. You may want to try other seasonings such as allspice, basil, dill, onions, and shallots, or sprinkle vinegar or low-sodium soy sauce in the cooking water.

Produce. Here's some conflicting information regarding pesticides that you might want to tuck into the forefront of your mind. According to the Food Marketing Institute, "The relationship between cancer and exposure to pesticides remains an issue with many unanswered questions." And the Food and Drug Administration reports, "the amounts we find in food are very low . . . and we believe . . . do not constitute a public health hazard."

To minimize potential risk:

- Rinse all produce thoroughly and, when possible, scrub fruits and vegetables with a brush. If possible, remove the skin.
- Discard the outer leaves of leafy vegetables.
- Choose in-season, locally grown products, which tend to have less pesticides than imported foods or foods grown far away from where they're sold.
- Vary the produce you eat.

Salt. The average American eats 20 times more salt than the daily requirement of ¼ teaspoon. Salt is an ingredient in soft drinks, fast foods, processed foods, cheese, and high-salt meats such as bacon, ham, sausage, frankfurters, and lunch meats. Try substituting herbs, spices, and lemon juice as flavoring.

Grains. For breakfast, lunch, snacks, and dinner, there is a variety of grains to choose from.

For breakfast, try these cereals: unprocessed oatmeal, amaranth cereal, brown rice and almond cereal by Kellogg's, NutriGrain Corn or Whole Wheat cereal, or millet cereal with berries. If you like breads, here are some suggestions: sprouted grain bread or toast, cornbread muffins, or oat bran muffins sweetened with fruit juice. And don't forget buckwheat pancakes—with natural Vermont maple syrup for a taste explosion.

Lunch choices include whole wheat pita bread sandwiches stuffed with a variety of you-name-it foods: garbanzo beans, tuna, bean sprouts, whatever you want. For other types of sandwiches, try five- or seven-grain bread, real rye, or whole wheat breads. (Avoid using commercial mayonnaise. It often contains sugar and oils that have gone rancid.)

For snacks, choose from brown rice cakes, perhaps spread with apple butter, almond butter, Sorrell Ridge jelly, or whatever you like. You might also try popcorn or whole wheat pretzels. And don't forget all the delicious whole-grain cookies sweetened with fruit juice!

Dinner can include oriental noodles such as udon, soba, or ramen, or whole wheat, buckwheat, artichoke, or spinach pasta. Use barley in soups or as a rice substitute and buckwheat as a side dish in kasha or as buckwheat crepes. Bulgur is good in cold salads or as a rice substitute. Use brown rice instead of white rice.

You've Done It!

You've now come to the end of the Body-Signal Program. But there's one final recommendation.

Go look in the mirror. What you'll see is an Instinctive Eater who responds to her Body Signals.

Congratulations!

You've just become one of the 4½ billion people who eat when they're hungry, stop when they're satisfied—and have *no* weight problem.

Index

Boldface references indicate tables.

Rodale Press, Inc., publishes PREVENTION, America's leading health magazine.
For information on how to order your subscription,
write to PREVENTION, Emmaus, PA 18098.